Healthy Living:
Alternative Health Solutions and their Impact on your Spiritual Nature

Richard Rosen

Those who do not find time every day for health must sacrifice a lot of time one day for illness.

(Sign in my holistic physician's office)

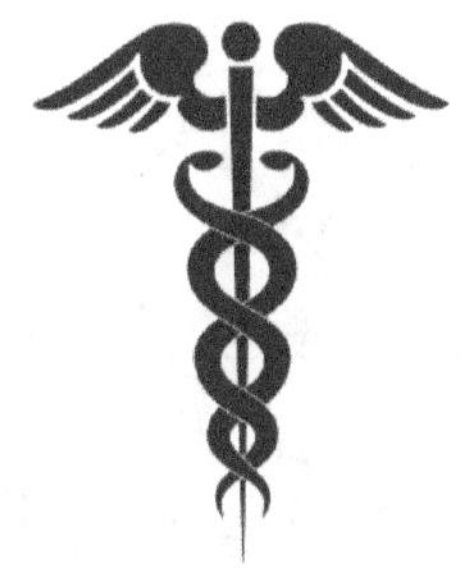

Let this not be said of you:

Ram Dass [a well-known spiritual teacher], 71, suffered a massive stroke…that resulted in long stays in the hospital and nursing home….(He) admitted that while he paid attention to his spiritual side, he often ignored his physical health. "I did not care for my body," he said. "I cared for my psychology and my soul, but I never cared for my body.[1]

ISBN-10: 1723423041
ISBN-13: 978-1723423048

My Books

www.LivingSpiritually.weebly.com

Life After Death: A step by step account of what happens next

Healthy Living: Alternative health solutions and their impact on your spiritual nature

Angelic Planetary Management: How the world got into its terrible condition and how we'll get out of it

Living Spiritually in a Practical World: How to attune yourself to divine guidance

God Speaking: Heavenly answers to earthly problems with life-altering decisions

The Divine Overcontrol of Civilization: Intelligent design and political, economic, social, and religious evolution

You can reach me at RichardRosen288@startmail.com.

What others have to say

Richard Rosen has gone over all the important facts that we need to know to stay healthy. Following his guidelines will help you obtain better health and happiness. Reading this book will save you years of searching for answers and put you on the right track to resolving your health concerns. Healthy Living embodies the body, mind, and spirit.

I finished reading your book Healthy Living. I give it an A+. It was easy to read, very clear, and, if followed, will save many lives. Thank you for caring about people; your book is a blessing to all of us.

I thoroughly enjoyed your new book. It was a very balanced approach in pointing out that the current material medical model, although important, is not the exclusive and only tool we have when dealing with health matters. Our belief in God or our spiritual nature, as well as natural holistic methods, is also of paramount importance as the book aptly details with excellent reference sources.

It's not like a huge, big novel that you have to read. Richard has it all right there in 70 or so pages.

A wonderful book that puts traditional medical care in proper perspective, and shows there is so much more available through alternative methods of holistic care, proper eating, and natural methods. Most importantly it stresses the mind, body, spiritual connection with God in the end always with us eternally. Excellent references for those interested in pursuing alternative practices not to the exclusion of traditional medicine but in complement. Highly recommended!

Saw an interview after reading the author's book and it reinforces just how important and valuable the material in this book is. The author looked healthy as a horse, which shows the proof is in the pudding!

I just picked it up again this morning and read a few chapters. It is such a simple book that imparts great wisdom. A treasure in a complicated world.

Contents

Preface

Most people have not experienced a live war zone where your life is at stake every moment. This applies to our health as well. Although this comparison may seem melodramatic, it is nevertheless true. Every moment of the day our health is in peril because we live in a toxic culture, one which pollutes the environment with abandon, one that has made a failed medical system into unassailable doctrine, one in which those in government, corporations, and even science so-called seek to silence alternative views. As on a battlefield with soldiers suffering grievous wounds, people anticipate chronic ill health and the miserable death that follows. But that need not be so as astutely recognized by this physician in 1929:

> (I am) thoroughly convinced that when this public fully realizes that all of its diseases are self-created, and to exactly the same extent self-controllable, the present fear of disease as a great and dangerous mystery will have passed, and health will be restored in the simple and effective ways.[2]

It is a shame that people invariably wait until they are afflicted by ill health before they search out why they are ailing. Such knowledge is best obtained when healthy, for then will you prevent disease by putting into practice what you have learned. But alas, few people study what it takes to remain strong and healthy. Instead they remain satisfied with superficial explanations from the medical establishment and unwittingly resolve only their symptoms.

Despite how dire the situation is, few people recognize its danger, although they are increasing in number. I believe the lifestyle change needed to counteract the peril to our health is so life-altering that many think to themselves, *I'll take my chances rather than deny myself the pleasures of indulging what I enjoy* (and spare myself the effort to learn).

I've written this book for those who are ready to turn their lives from chronic ill health to optimal wellness. I hope you number yourself among them.

* * *

Because each of us is unique, the suggestions I make will not apply to everyone. As I grow older and learn more, I adjust my health regimen, and so will you. I hope you will be inspired by the things that work for me, that they stimulate your thinking, for the answers to your problems lie within. True answers always come from within, not from outside sources, not even from well-meaning people of great experience. Haven't you noticed the contradictory opinions that confound so many issues? Rather, learn to make up your own mind that it may be said of you, *There goes one healthy human being.*

Note on the use of gender pronouns. *Man* and its pronouns are used to denote a human being or mankind. So ladies, please don't take offense; and men, don't get a swelled head.

How did I arrive at my philosophy of healthy living? We each develop a personal philosophy of living that informs our acting and thinking. The source which has most influenced how I comprehend reality is *The Urantia Book.* Along with soul growth, strength of character, and comprehending the world, has come knowing who I am and my purpose for living (not bad!) I discovered the Urantia book in 1985, and it became my compass through which to navigate life. For those unfamiliar with it and would like to know more, I suggest looking at the table of contents and read what draws your attention, what you would like to know more about (https://archive.urantiabook.org/newbook/index.html) or look at an overview: https://urantiabook.org/the-urantia-book/overview).

Introduction

We each have a life journey that depends on the smooth working of the various levels of our being, one of which is our health. The physical body forms the base of the pyramid of the whole person; it is the material part of man. Mind and spirit comprise the other two levels. The three domains must operate in harmony for a person to be whole, fulfilled, happy, and successful.

Unfortunately, there is often a disconnect between being healthy in body, harmonious in mind, and attuned to spirit. And so the purpose of this book is to:

- optimize health so the material body can serve as the foundation on which rests a sound mind and a spiritual nature;
- point out the current state of ill health and the reasons for it;
- take control and become beautiful specimens of manhood and womanhood—whatever our age!

I am a believer that most difficulties are of our own making. But what about those things beyond our control, such as heredity and the accidents of time? Fortunately, even these can be made the best of. We create the environment in which we live and our health improves or deteriorates accordingly.

We each need to take control of our health by making our own medical decisions with the input from practitioners who share our viewpoint, all the while researching those things needful to maintain a sound and healthy body. Here is an example of taking control:

> I had been taking hormones to balance out things. I took blood tests for my next appointment and it turned out my medical specialist did not include certain hormones for testing. I had relied on him to include them. In his busyness he did not and so I had to take another blood test.
>
> It made me realize that it is my responsibility to check everything, not only to ensure what should be present is there, but also to make suggestions for other things that may be appropriate. Moreover, I recognized that as I gain more knowledge that I need not consult with him on all things, having gained the wisdom to know when I could do things on my own. A doctor should be a trusted

professional with whom you share ideas and value his expertise and counsel. But he had better respect your point of view about alternative health solutions and not discount them because they are not countenanced by medical authorities.

Health is innate. We are designed so we do not need interventions to maintain it, except for accidents and life-threatening infections. However, institutionalized medicine cannot help but result in debilitation. As with everything else in life, it's our decision to control our health. But it requires courageous and independent thinking. It takes research, willingness to think beyond what's commonly accepted as healthcare, and the courage to make decisions that may run counter to mainstream medical advice.

This can begin at any age and at any state of health. The healing mechanisms that deal with disease and accident are effective in proportion to how we live in harmony with the material laws of health. It's marvelous how the body is programmed to heal itself, to right the ship of wellbeing and chart a new course. We determine our own health for good or bad—no one else.

These are the main things that determine health in my view:

- Nutrition
- Movement and exercise
- Minimized exposure to environmental toxins
- Correct posture
- Resolving stress
- Knowledge of alternative medical solutions coupled with an awareness of the limitations and dangers of conventional medicine. "The entirety of traditional medicine is mostly aimed at alleviating the symptoms associated with a disease, while leaving the continued progression of the disease itself unaddressed."[3]

THE HEALTHY LIFESTYLE

Live in harmony with nature

My mantra for making lifestyle decisions has become, *How does non-industrial man live?* That is because the debilitating diseases that plague us today were unknown 150 years ago. Back then, waterborne illness from a lack of hygiene was prevalent, such as cholera, typhoid, and dysentery. That is largely gone, at least in first world countries, but replaced with chemicalized food and environmental toxins that destroy the body's terrain and its innate ability to heal. Here's what I mean:

- Non-industrial man lives in harmony with nature. Recognizing how our modern environment is changing radically, it is essential that we learn how to support living in a natural environment.
- They are outdoors and in sunlight many hours. They arise with the sun and go to bed not long after it sets. Our health will substantially improve if we live according to circadian rhythm; our internal clock is regulated by sunlight and directs the processes of the body 24/7.
- Nighttime lighting is gentle: candle, lamp oil, firelight, moonlight. We can approach the ideal by using incandescent bulbs or LEDs that have reduced blue light and flicker. (I buy mine at www.waveformlighting.com, in particular, the 1700K Flicker-Free A19 bulb).
- Their feet touch the earth. Thus grounded they soak up electrons which enhance mitochondria function. We can spend time barefoot on the ground or grounding mats indoors.
- Non-industrial man moves throughout the day accomplishing the chores of living. We can do likewise by movement and exercise.
- They eat food that is local and in season.
- Being in nature is calming: it reduces stress.
- They are masters of their level of technology, not its slave.
- They drink water untainted by chemical additions and uncontaminated by industrial pollutants.

- Their environment is void of electro-smog (non-native electromagnetic fields (nmEMF)), such as WiFi and electrical wiring. I know it sounds impossible to avoid, but it can be substantially minimized. I have done so (learn about it at www.safespaceprotection.com).
- They heal themselves with the "tree of life, whose leaves were for the 'healing of the nations' ...."4 This represents natural medicine: plants, herbs, natural teas, tinctures, homeopathy, medicinals, and energy medicine—healing modalities evolved over thousands of years that our great-grandparents knew and used.
- They are attuned to their bodies; they listen. They use their innate intuition; they have not so focused on the analytical side of their brains that the intuitive side has atrophied.

There is a science that encompasses living in harmony with nature: Quantum Biology. You can learn more at Carrie B. Wellness, https://www.carriebwellness.com/. It is where I learned and participated in a community of like-minded people who are reclaiming their birthright and restoring their health to how God intended it to be.

Treat disease in cooperation with nature

William Howard Hay, a medical doctor, wrote in 1929, "Now, after twenty-four years of treatment of disease wholly without drugs or surgery..., (my) treatment is a let-alone plan, letting feeding alone, letting medicine alone, letting everything alone that the patient does not crave. Nature never fails to restore to health the body thus let alone, usually far better health than before the illness."5

He went on to say, "(...my prescription...for the symptoms of disease...was harmful and suppressive of Nature's efforts to right the internal wrongs in her own way."6

Become your own doctor

I have become my own doctor. My goal is to extricate myself from the medical complex by practicing preventative healthcare, by *being* healthy.

I used to have a long-term relationship with a local physician whom I would see every two years for a checkup. He's well respected in the community and local hospital, so he was the person I wanted in my corner should I have needed conventional care. He respected my effort to control my health and was aware of my alternative medical practitioners. Therefore, not having an annual exam was all right with him. (When he first told his staff to schedule me in two years, they were surprised, it being the only time it had happened.) I concluded our relationship because the local hospital was bought by a hospital chain and local doctors no longer could visit their patients and be responsible for their care.

As with everything else in life, we evolve in our understanding of what it means to live healthy. What we know today is less than what we will know tomorrow. Therefore, I find myself either tweaking or altering my health regimen as I learn more.

> I entered "the path…of learning about my body, what interacts with my body, and to give the body what it needs to heal and operate at its maximum." (Michael Stroka, president of the American Nutrition Association)

With the poor ethics practiced by many businesses today, companies will often manufacture health products and deliver health services they either know are unhealthy or they choose to remain willfully ignorant of in the pursuit of profit. Think of the tobacco industry; then apply the same mindset to what I'd dare say is every industry to some degree.

> Pharmaceutical and meat companies are using similar tactics to the cigarette industry, in an attempt to confuse consumers and hold off regulation, despite the fact that the rapidly growing risk of antimicrobial resistance is one of the biggest health risks of our time.[7]

Alternative medicine that promotes non-conventional wellness solutions has risen in protest. The same is happening in other industries as well, but generally it is the smaller business that chooses ethical solutions. Once a company has lost the ethical compass and drive of its founders, the widespread mentality of profit above all takes hold. Vitiated products and service invariably follow.

It's wise—no, it's crucial—to research alternative views about wellness and health issues you are dealing with. It is essential to have sources who are integris and refuse to conform to the conventional medical narrative. *Continual* learning about medical issues and healthy lifestyle determine if you will recover from current medical issues and go on to live a healthy life. The reality of a situation must be recognized together with the wisdom and courage to act.

In my experience, the effort is too great for most people and they fall back on the rationalization that disease and disability are inevitable and there's little you can do about them; failing and dying miserably is part of life. Not true! Rather, there are few conditions that cannot be healed, and those can often be made better.

These sites are some of my sources of health information. They differ markedly from mainstream sources and standardized medical thinking.

- Weston A Price Foundation https://www.westonaprice.org/The best site I have found for practical information on healthy living.

- Dr. Mercola's Censored Library https://www.mercola.com/ or https://takecontrol.substack.com/ He presents essential information on many topics.

- The Forgotten Side of Medicine https://www.midwesterndoctor.com/ This doctor exposes pharmaceutical corruption and discusses remarkable therapies once practiced but now lost to time. These are in-depth articles, so be prepared to learn a lot.

- Children's Health Defense https://childrenshealthdefense.org/ Their mission is to restore and protect the health of children, but includes practical information for adults." (not a main resource for me, but a valuable one nonetheless)

- The Rowen Report https://drrowen.substack.com/ This Doctor talks about his experiences with therapies that alternative medical practitioners use with remarkable results, how to remain healthy, and related political issues.

- Doctor Tom Cowan https://drtomcowan.com/ His mantra is to "question everything." He has arrived at a "new biology," a way to comprehend health, to which I subscribe.

- Carrie Bennett https://www.carriebwellness.com/ I characterize Carrie's work as how to cooperate with your body and with nature to live a life of harmony. I learned much and implemented it.

Find a knowledgeable alternative medical practitioner you trust and feel good to. Use him or her regularly and proactively (although the end goal is to become knowledgeable and experienced so you have "become your own doctor"). Make it your business to allocate the time and to find the resources to keep you healthy—your life depends on it.

Carrie Bennett, a quantum biology healer, puts it well:

Healing is a natural state once we learn to be in resonance with nature. I'm simply here as a guide to that resonance, not a medical professional or your health savior. I enjoy working the most with individuals who believe healing is within their power.

I know you are likely coming here because you have already tried many things to heal you and/or your family and you're hoping I and quantum biology will be your "fix," but the honest reality is that healing doesn't typically happen in a single session (or even three, or even with a single practitioner). Even though circadian and quantum biology can make massive improvements in your health quickly, chronic illness does not solve itself overnight; living within all of the challenges of modernity means that being fully "healed" is a true challenge.

Take control and experiment

The prevalent way of thinking relies on government and professionals to provide healthcare. Control is thereby abdicated and given to others. It is crucial for optimal health to develop the mindset that health is foremost individual responsibility. This enables a person to take control and avoid succumbing to the awe of medical credentials and its medical advice. Here is the experience of a registered nurse:

> During that visit, had I been one iota less aware, knowledgeable, and experienced, it could have quickly turned disastrous, both for what they would have done with excessive, unneeded testing and treatments, and a bloated billing.
>
> That one visit, that lasted only a few hours of nothing, could have bankrupted us, as it has for many. Ah, well...it's a great refresher course to motivate me to do better on my own! How glad I am not to have been unconscious so I could direct my care and limit theirs![8]

Hear what doctors have to say, and then analyze, evaluate, and decide for yourself. Beware: until you are confident in your view of medicine, it is not easy to resist the authority of a doctor. Here's my experience:

> During a medical exam there were some issues that came up with my heart and it was recommended that I see a cardiologist. Unexpectedly, and to my surprise, testing revealed that part of my heart had died. Wow!
>
> I figured out the cause. I was gluten intolerant for many years before it was diagnosed. Among other things, it caused intestinal permeability or leaky gut (food material enters the bloodstream) which caused inflammation. Inflammation is associated with heart disease.
>
> A heart catheterization was strongly advised and it made sense to undergo the procedure and see what else was happening. Further surprise—the test discovered not only the 100% blockage that cut off the blood supply to the dead portion of my heart, there were also two

blockages of 80% and smaller ones of 50-60%. And I had no symptoms.

Before undergoing the procedure I researched alternatives to stents and the drug therapy that accompanies them. I realize now that I should have consulted with my holistic physician, but I didn't. Everything was rushed. Live and learn.

After the procedure I was prescribed three drugs, and my cardiologist told me they were for life. As with all pharmaceuticals, I knew they are toxic to some degree. I researched extensively. I consulted with my holistic physician and he referred me to a naturopath physician who specialized in IV therapy. After extensive testing of vitamin, mineral, and other health markers, I underwent intravenous vitamins and minerals and CheZone therapy (chelation and ozone developed by Frank Shallenberger) for six weeks and customized daily supplementation that continued afterward. I could tell immediately that it was working because a crippling back issue improved after each session until it was gone. As for my heart, I could do increasingly more yard work and exercise.

Meanwhile, I stayed on the drugs for five months because drug therapy is essential for a period of time once you have stents. And then I stopped the pills. Is there a risk I might be wrong? Of course. But there is documented evidence of people declining and dying prematurely from these drugs. As with many drugs, conclusions vary widely between conventional and alternative medicine clinicians and researchers. I weighed everything and made my decision. Here is *some* of that evidence from which I decided to stop taking these pharmaceuticals:

- One of the drugs prescribed was a blood thinner, a generic of Plavix, together with aspirin. The conclusion of my research was that they increase the risk of death, double the risk of gastrointestinal bleeding,; and more than double fatal hemorrhaging. You can read details in the endnote.[9]
- Another drug prescribed was a statin, a generic of Lipitor. Here is a summary of the dangers:

"There is evidence showing that statins may actually make your heart health worse and only appear effective due to statistical deception. Statins deplete your body of CoQ10, inhibit synthesis of vitamin K2, and reduce the production of ketone bodies. Statins increase your risk of serious diseases including cancer, diabetes, neurodegenerative diseases, musculoskeletal disorders and cataracts."[10] It can also cause transient amnesia.[11]

At the next appointment with my cardiologist I told him I had stopped the medications. From his reaction I suspect that I may have been the first patient who on his own researched and made the decision to disregard his pharmaceuticals-for-life instruction. I say this because his first question was, "Did someone advise you to do this?" When I told him no, and after he soundly warned me of the dangers, I remained firm in my resolve. But I thought, *How difficult it is for people to disregard a doctor's strongly worded advice.*

Here is an example of an individual who took control of his medical life.

I've been through the mill with endocrine illnesses and countless operations. Consequently, I do not follow doctors' advice—I am an independent thinker and wiser now!

I like to experiment, trying new supplements. Then I carefully listen to my body and learn how it responds. Also, I like to think that my body, being very sensitive, is my lab for this life, and I trust how it responds.

I never stop asking questions until I feel that something rings true for me. I am in the basket of too hard a case, and doctors scratch their head. But pain and outcomes have taught me how each of us human beings on this planet is unique in his character, biology and physiology, hence my renewed positive outlook on life, just as it should be.

Fortunately, people are becoming increasingly aware and taking control of their health as this person had.

To sum it up, take control of your health and take back your power from medical professionals. In other words, *become your own doctor.*

Damage to your health is reversible

The body is designed for self-healing for which we must take responsibility for it to be effective. We do this by recognizing the true cause of dis-ease. Lifestyle changes must be made that stop what caused the problem, which allows the wonderfully designed healing mechanism of the body to do its work.

There are numerous stories of intractable diseases that have been resolved when conventional medicine failed. But it's usually after exhausting conventional solutions that the person educates himself and tries alternative therapies. If you are dealing with such a situation, you may want to read Doctor Andrew Weil's book, *Spontaneous Healing : How to Discover and Embrace Your Body's Natural Ability to Maintain and Heal Itself.*

What to eat

The way in which we commune with nature on a daily basis is through the food we eat. It's truly amazing and beautiful and just harmonious the way in which food is designed to work in our body. We need to make healthier food choices. (Dr. Michael Murray, N.D.)

Americans have grown fat—obese for many. People eat more than is needed. This reflects a spiritual state that is not at all appealing: people ignore their spiritual nature in favor of their animal appetites. A nutritionist explains the effect that food has on becoming all you are capable of becoming:

The norm is to be overweight, fatigued, and do only what is needed to get by, and so getting by becomes the benchmark.　Food has everything to do with this.　You become what you put in your mouth, and your food environment [the culture of food] is about profit and pleasure, not about making you the best you can be.

You can't reach your optimum self with a sub-optimal vessel.　You will give away your dreams and follow [what everyone else does].　You will not be…the positive change God intended.　It is hard to do great things when you have the burden of a tired, depressed, unmotivated vessel; this…become your focus.　Food has everything to do with this.[12]

Our bodies require less to live on than we now consume. It's healthier to eat less.

An elderly couple told my wife, Eve, and me years ago that they eat only breakfast and lunch. The thought was astounding. No dinner? That's the American way: breakfast, lunch, dinner—and snacks between. They said they found it sufficient for their age, having slowed down. And they looked good. We followed their example.

What did our healthy ancestors eat?

This post from a Weston A Price Foundation (www.westonaprice.org) member says it well:

In my 20s my energy and focus were dwindling so I began asking the question what should I eat? I found many suggestions but could not decide which made the most sense. I eliminated junk food, I eliminated meat, and eventually all animal foods after reading a book on one person's ideas about healthy eating. But I was not convinced it was the best and what proof was there?

Finally, I learned about observations made of people who were healthy and eating the foods that they had learned about from their parents, grandparents and back for generations. They were healthy and were eating according to the real practices of their healthy ancestors, not a recent theory about diet.

I learned about this from a conversation and a book by Sally Fallon Morell (*Nourishing Traditions®: The Cookbook that Challenges Politically Correct Nutrition and the Diet Dictocrats*). This information changed my life. I have more energy in my 50s than I had in my 20s!" (Kathy K.)

Cook food at home

While it may seem unrealistic in this ultra-busy society we inhabit, I'm convinced it is the only way to achieve a healthy diet. And when the value of a goal is truly recognized, it will be achieved.

Here are two reasons why preparing your own food is so important. I have learned to do so and enjoy it. (This is from an article by *A Midwestern Doctor*.[13])

1. "The less processed food you eat, the healthier you will be.

2. "Better quality ingredients equate to better health.

"In most cases, both of these are only possible to achieve if you cook food at home, so I believe Christmas dinners represent an ideal time to learn those skills from relatives already well versed in them (or practice them yourselves) rather than purchasing premade meals."

Avoid dangerous foods

Eating mostly whole foods, such as root vegetables, fruit, and nuts, is best. Meat and fish are fine, provided meat is grass fed and fish is wild caught. Otherwise, they will harm you.

Contamination of meat by heavy metals, veterinary drugs and pesticides is a problem which the U.S. government has for the most part ignored. And while bacterial contaminants can be killed by cooking, chemical residues stay in the meat.

Sick dairy cows are given medications to help them recover, but if it appears an animal will die, it's often sold to a slaughterhouse as quickly as possible, in time to kill it before it dies.

…hormones, antibiotics and pesticides are part of most supermarket meat….[14]

How do you find healthy food and local farms? Here are two sources: http://www.5thbranch.com/find-local-organic-farm-near/ https://www.localharvest.org/. And ask around where the farms are, such as a farmers market. Get to know your farmers.

I recommend this book that will tell you how to navigate the grocery store and where to buy real food. A remarkable healing journey is recounted.

BEYOND LABELS: A Doctor and a Farmer Conquer Food Confusion One Bite at a Time. Joel Salatin and Sina McCullough. https://www.youtube.com/watch?v=ErOnc1AfW6c (Interview)

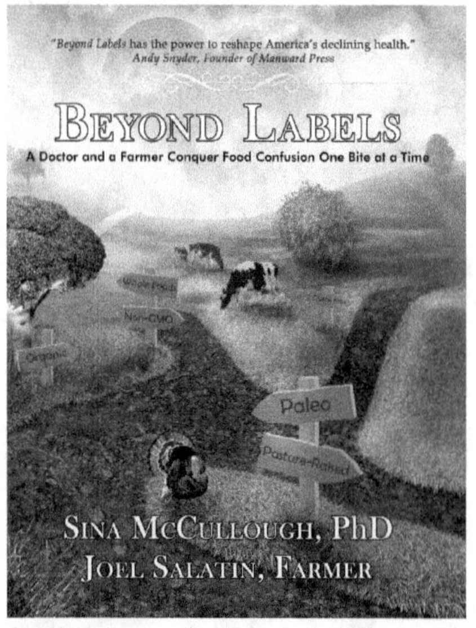

Beware the deceitfulness of self-serving marketing. Business, government, and self-interest groups are sophisticated enough to use marketing sleight-of-hand. To be fair, the advertising and marketing industry has to be admired. How clever and effective they are in persuading people to do things against their best interest. Remember, this age is profit dominated: bottom line above all, even to the ill health and death of millions. Not only is truth not valued, it is a hindrance to their objectives. Think of the tobacco industry that knowingly falsified its marketing and hid the truth about its death delivery products to the devastation of millions of lives and harm to society. This kind of deceit extends to every aspect of society; our semi-civilization often lives by the maxim that the end justifies the means.

It behooves us therefore to be wise as serpents when dealing with food companies that legally falsify their health claims to increase sales, pharmaceutical companies that knowingly push toxic drugs to fatten their wallets, politicians who cleverly tell you whatever it takes to get elected—and so on.

> Legally prescribed drugs kill hundreds of thousands of people a year. (Dr. Joseph Mercola)

It is rare for someone to tell the truth about his product and recommend its use only when others will truly benefit. Unfortunately, the attitude that prevails these days is, *What's good for me is better than what's good for you*. Here is an example of such selfishness:

> There is an annual maintenance cost associated with the software I had sold. I was careful that my customers knew what the cost would be so they could factor it into their purchase decision. My associate, on the other hand, designedly refused to volunteer anything about maintenance lest he lose the sale. He told me, "I say whatever it takes to get them to take out their credit card."

It bears repeating, "Be wise as serpents but harmless as doves."

The best food label is a farmer you can trust

Exercise

Exercise is more than your backup plan; it should be front and center in your daily life. Effective fitness habits play a primary and foundational role in your healthy metabolism and disease prevention. (Dr. Richard Maurer)[15]

To put a number on it, I would say that exercise and movement is 30-40 % of the health equation. It must be consistent if it is to be effective. There are many forms; choose those you enjoy for you are more likely to do them.

Exercise changes over time as your body requires different forces acting on it to maintain strength, stability, performance, and health. I had a set of exercises using bands for several years (and I walk daily at a fast gait for 20+ minutes; it's my time to commune with Spirit as well). My naturopath doctor told me I need to get my heart moving more and to incorporate cardio. So for the first time in my life I departed from my best effort collection of exercises and hired a personal trainer to customize a set of exercises. Wow! What an eye-opener!

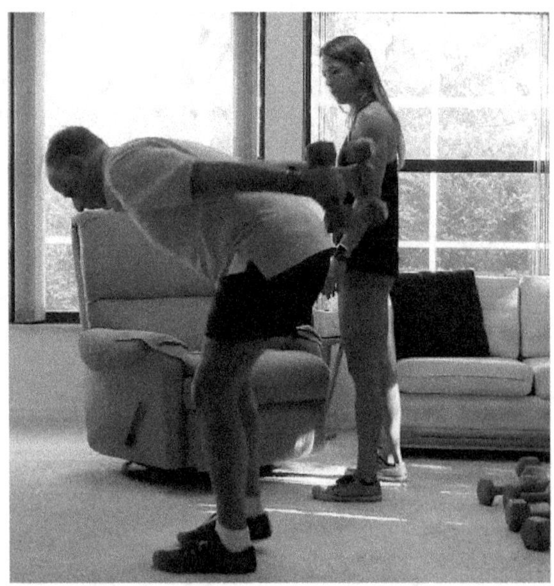

As I said, things change and we need to be flexible and sensitive enough to reflect those changes in new ways of doing things.

One last thing, on occasion I am not up to it; so I've learned to listen to my body, respect what it's saying, and not force it.

Stress

Stress not dealt with properly creates havoc with the body. This is where the mind-body connection becomes apparent in a negative way. But stress has a positive side; it is needed for growth.

We are living through more change in the last 100 years than in thousands of years before—and in these later decades it is even more rapid. Change requires adaptation which causes stress. When handled properly it serves as a goad to our inherently lazy animal natures to adapt and grow—at least until we have mastered the art of self-motivated progress. Change stimulates us to achieve physical health, intellectual clarity, emotional maturity, and spiritual insight.

I handle stress foremost by stepping aside, seeing it from a high vantage point, one I call cosmic or spiritual. I work to remain personally uninvolved so my emotions do not cloud my judgment. But I'm careful not to remain insensitive and aloof. Empathy and compassion are a must. I reach into the wisdom I've accumulated and seek the counsel of others when warranted to discern how best to handle a situation. A guiding principle is to maximize the good to all involved that would result from the action I take.

With so many things stressing us, many evil in nature, it wears us out on all levels of our being: physical, mental-emotional, and spiritual. These energies need to be replenished, which requires intelligent recreation and relaxation.

Being a unified personality is crucial to handle stress well. It is reflected in the balance of the material and the spiritual. The resulting harmony marshals the resources of a together personality, one of maturity and goodness that is guided by wisdom.

Toxins

We have become a chemicalized society. What I mean is that the chemical industry has become ubiquitous in the products we eat, put on our skin, and breathe. Chronic end-of-life diseases that plague most elderly people in developed countries are in large part caused by decades of ingesting chemicals and exposure to a toxic environment. I'm convinced that Alzheimer's has its origin in this accumulated toxicity. Mix in a little more monosodium glutamate (MSG)? How about a wee bit of yellow dye? Ugh!

I asked my alternative medical practitioner about a skin lotion, showing him the ingredients. There were more than a dozen chemical formulations, most of which could not be pronounced easily. He took one look and said, "As a rule of thumb, if you cannot pronounce it, don't eat it or put it on your skin." (Ladies, watch those cosmetics!) And neither would I breathe it, which means from such sources as cleaning supplies, secondhand smoke, or air polluted cities that you can avoid visiting—and certainly think twice about living there.

Tap water has an abundance of contaminants, regardless of meeting regulatory requirements. Having a water filter is crucial, and it needs to be a top-quality one. The one I recommend is AquaPerform from Multipure (https://www.multipure.com/products/drinking-water-systems/aquaperform).

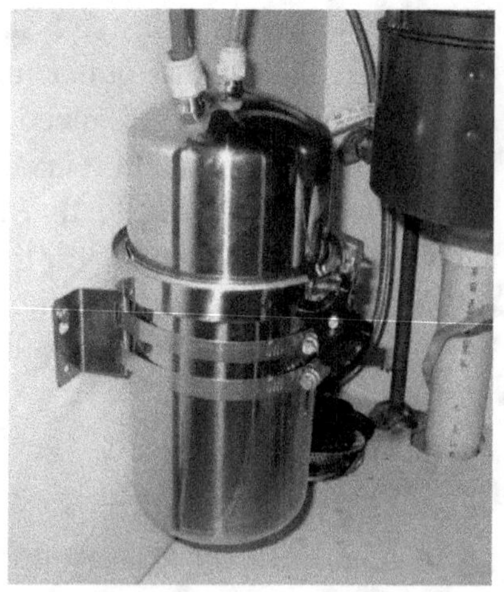

Countertop and less expensive alternatives: www.ClearlyFiltered.com and www.epicwaterfilters.com.

Beware of these dangers

I was reluctant to include this list of pervasive health dangers lest I overwhelm those new to thinking about health differently than what is generally accepted. I know it took me some time to believe these things were true and refuse or reduce their presence in my life. I am healthier for it. I include references after each entry to make it easier to see what they're about.

- vaccination https://www.nvic.org/
- electromagnetic frequency fields (EMF): wireless technologies such as cell phones and Bluetooth https://buildingbiologyinstitute.org/; https://childrenshealthdefense.org/emr/emf-wireless-health-impacts https://www.safespaceprotection.com/
- gluten https://grainstorm.com/pages/modern-wheat https://www.drperlmutter.com/focus-area/gluten-free/ https://www.glutenfreesociety.org/about-us-2/
- microwave ovens https://www.safespaceprotection.com/news-and-info/microwave-oven-dangers/ and https://www.westonaprice.org/health-topics/debunking-the-myth-that-microwave-ovens-are-harmless/#gsc.tab=0
- mercury fillings https://mercuryfreedentistry.net/
- fluoridated water http://fluoridealert.org/
- genetically engineered foods (GMO) https://responsibletechnology.org/;
- artificial sweeteners https://drjockers.com/artificial-sweeteners/
- childhood trauma—Your thoughts and feelings, your ideas and emotions, must be healed from the traumas of childhood for your body to be healthy. Otherwise these negative energies will continue to affect your health. A practitioner of this method uncovered a deep-seated trauma in me. This is the book in his waiting room that I purchased and read: *Good News For People Who Hurt and It's N.E.A.T.* by Lou Ann Dickerson Hall https://www.amazon.com/gp/product/0970703341

The value of disease

I recount this story as an example of how an apparently insurmountable problem can be a turning point of leaving the apparent security of consensus medicine to follow your own leading. This experience carries over to other areas of life as well.

I began learning about health, in particular alternative health solutions, in the early 90s when I was forced to deal with digestive issues. The medical folks at the University of Connecticut teaching hospital couldn't figure out the problem after they took a stab at tropical parasites. Coincidentally, I found an alternative health practitioner (my first exposure) and he quickly diagnosed the problem—lactose intolerance; I couldn't digest milk products. Well hallelujah! As simple as that! That's when I began reading books by Dr. Andrew Weil, a well-regarded practitioner of integrative medicine. I have continued learning these many years.

This is an example of personal growth that can result from ill health, even devastating disease. Here is an email I received:

Richard, I was a caretaker to my parents (Dad for 4 years and Mom for 6) every other month in another state. My sister (who also lived in a different state than our parents) and I alternated months. Another sister pitched-in when she could. We ALL grew together in unconditional love and support.

I felt that my parents' condition was actually a way for their souls to evolve. Dad viewed the world from a very happy place. His glass was always half full. He was creative, musical and artistic. Toward the end of his life, he lost his vision and hearing, forcing him to change the way he related to the world. Meanwhile, Mom, who was always tense and controlling, suffered (I do not use this term lightly) from Alzheimer's disease. She was a giver who finally learned to receive—Alzheimer's disease gave her no other option.

When my parents started their physical decline, the dynamics of their relationship changed, and Dad's last four years were the happiest years in their marriage. Dad reoriented Mom and took control of their relationship, and Mom gently guided Dad, explaining what he couldn't see or hear—quite a change from the hurried, annoyed demeanor he was used to interacting with. They evolved spiritually until the end of their lives—truly the silver lining of the proverbial dark cloud.

I would have to say, the entire family benefitted, including our parents' great-granddaughter. Our Mom went with us to pick her up from school every day. This child formed a very deep connection to her great-grandmother. She could always figure out how to connect with Mom. Her schoolteacher told her she was very lucky to have support from so many people who love her! I believe her great-grandmother may have loved her most.

This experience taught us all the blessing of unconditional love. I would not change this for anything and would dearly love to have our beloved parents back to continue enriching our lives.

This novelist dramatized the concept:

Financial losses changed him in many ways. He became gentler. *And his illness brought out still more gentleness* [emphasis mine]. Doctor Warburton once said he wouldn't deprive any man or woman of the opportunities of a long-drawn-out last sickness. I know what he meant now. It was a second chance for us all—for me, for each of the children, and for Rupert too.[16]

ALTERNATIVE MEDICINE

An epidemic of chronic ill health now affects not only those who are in their final years but also children and young adults in their beginning and early years. And we as a people continue to grow sicker and sicker. Obviously, what the conventional medical establishment offers is not working. For most people it takes a lot of time, effort, and money exhausting conventional medicine and themselves before seriously considering alternatives. It is for this reason I am telling you about alternate solutions to healing and optimizing your health so you avoid getting sick and becoming diseased. This is often referred to as alternative medicine, holistic medicine, complementary and alternative medicine (CAM), and integrative medicine.

I began my education in alternative medicine in the early 90s by reading books by Dr. Andrew Weil. From him I learned that foundational to healthy living is recognizing that the body is designed to heal itself; we just need to stay out of the way by removing the conditions that prevent it, whether from what we eat or the environment or our mind and emotions.

There is a large array of alternative health solutions, enough to become bewildered; which do you choose? Each lays out a path to health. Each reaches the peak from a different side of the mountain. Each of us must decide which solutions align best with who we are. They all ascend to the same height, of not merely good, but optimal health. But remember always, underlying them all is living aligned with nature.

What follows are health solutions with which I have personal experience. There are many more. As with everything, it's crucial to determine what makes sense for *you*, what fits your unique array of physical needs. I include the experience of others in my research. It provides the authority of authenticity that balances the scientific and marketing claims of health solutions and products. I have found that clinical experience trumps scientific research.

Supplements

My view of supplementation has changed. I used to think it was essential because of the depletion of the soil. Now I recognize that if your food is grown in *healthy* soil by farmers you trust along with ethical distributors and retailers, you should be able to reduce or eliminate them. Nonetheless, supplements have a place when your life is not centered around food integrity.

Many people now recognize the toxicity of petrochemical drugs and seek to avoid them by substituting vitamins, minerals, and herbs. They think they are safer because they are natural, which is not altogether true. I am an example of having a serious autoimmune disease because of supplementation; I learned the hard way, which is often the case with us humans.

When it's all said and done, you cannot fix dietary error and lifestyle with supplementation. Supplements will not provide the benefits of food, sunlight, and movement—a lifestyle aligned with nature. "The more nutrient dense your diet, the fewer processed foods you eat, the closer you are to nature—the better off you are!"

Keep in mind that supplementation is for specific deficiencies and should cease when they have been remedied. Taking supplements beyond the immediate need causes the body to downregulate the ability to absorb the supplement (tachyphylaxis). You end up taking supplements and they no longer have value–or they even work against you. For example, vitamin D from sunlight has dozens of metabolites that act like stem cells in that they go wherever needed. This is in contrast to vitamin D3 supplementation which has only one pathway from the liver. You can learn more in this video: *Put down the Vitamin D supplements—you could be ruining your health!* https://www.youtube.com/watch?v=CqiQ7zyWSR4

Beware of so-called experts. Not infrequently they have differing and even contradictory views. How about common sense as shared here:

> This super complicated article basically says what my…mother had me do when I was a little girl. Play outside, eat whole foods, get fresh air and sunshine, make friends.

Sounds like the answer is pretty simple. Get off these damn phones, go for a long hike out in nature with a good dog, enjoy the company of other individuals actually engaged in life, eat real food, sit in the sun, play an instrument.

What baffles me is how information changes. With that said, I am in the 4th quarter of my life and have decided what's important for my health. It's really not what you eat, it's what you don't eat. Eat real food, grass fed, wild caught, pasture raised, all organic. Drink and bathe in clean water. Lift heavy stuff a few times a week, move every day, practice your balance on a regular basis. To your health!

When do you actually need to supplement your food?

Foremost is to be in touch with how you are feeling. Something off? Think about what you did or ate prior to feeling discomfort or disharmony. Make a change and over several days see if it makes a difference. And this could include taking a supplement. For example, in dealing with a heart issue, I had discovered Strophanthus Seed Extract, which has a significant impact on heart issues. I had been taking it for a while, and then experimented with stopping and seeing if there was an effect. And there was within a couple of days! So I resumed. You can read more about it here: *Strophanthus: "The Gift From Paradise"*
https://drtomcowan.com/blogs/blog/strophanthus-the-gift-from-paradise

For a more analytical approach, you can determine which supplements are needed with a nutritional assessment from an experienced health professional. A reader of my book wrote to me: "I continue to stay vigilant with my health, paying for my own screenings and additional testing; it is worth the money." While you can purchase labs directly from various online sites, interpretation requires experience, without which deciding what to do is like buying a pig in the poke.

Supplements have a cost to them, as well as paying the practitioner to evaluate what you need. He will recommend quality brands that cost more because so many are junk. My doctor told me it is better to halve a quality supplement if needed to meet your budget rather than take a poor one. I view the cost of supplements as an investment in health that will not only yield a superior quality of life but also substantially reduce medical costs by avoiding short-term illness and chronic disease. The bulk of spending will be getting initially assessed and follow up practitioner reviews. In a year or so the cost should diminish because either only maintenance will be needed or, better yet and the goal, you will no longer need them.

The supplement industry

Unfortunately, the supplement industry has its share of snazzy marketing whizzes with inferior products. I have come to distrust the glitz that cleverly urges each supplement as the best thing since sliced bread.

In a study conducted by ConsumerLab.com, researchers tested 11 brands of echinacea products and found out that only four of them contained the actual flower. The rest didn't meet the measurements stated in the packaging labels and, even worse, some of them didn't even contain echinacea at all! [17]

In the chart below are some of the manufacturers I have confidence in. I eliminated the ones that had been privately owned and begun by individuals who had a genuine desire to help others, but were purchased by pharmaceutical companies, private equity groups, and big business. Greed is the mantra not health as related in this example by my local supplement store. Dave told me that he had been selling a product for sleep that contained a well absorbed magnesium formulation. But a customer pointed out that it had been replaced by cheaper and less suitable form of magnesium in the year since it had been purchased. You can read more about it in this article: *The 14 Mega-Corporations That Own Your Supplement Brands* (2018) https://drnealsmoller.com/rant/the-14-mega-corporations-that-own-your-supplement-brand/

Cautions

"The solutions to your health problems in the traditional Western allopathic model of health and most functional or naturopathic models of health look primarily at what pill or supplement you might take to alleviate your symptoms and change your biochemistry. Low in magnesium? Take a magnesium supplement. Lacking in Vitamin D? Take a D3 supplement. High cholesterol? Take a statin.

"Since this doesn't change the underlying mechanisms driving your biochemistry to behave a certain way, it means you stay stuck taking pills or supplements and going through medical testing for a lot, if not the rest, of your life, continuing to check on the biochemical status of your body—like whether you have enough potassium or if your stomach lining is inflamed."[18]

"Big Ag and Big Pharma have now become Big Supplement, profiting off the nutrient gaps their own food system created. But your body was made for real, bioavailable nutrients from real food. It's time to ditch a long list of synthetic band-aids and get back to what matters."[19] This video short explains:
https://www.youtube.com/shorts/aDS2Bo_qNYk

"[What] I've found so challenging in the health field is knowing whether something I see supportive evidence and testimonials for actually works, as on one hand, many do, but I've also seen countless examples where it didn't, and then realized most of the "evidence" I saw for it had been artificially created (e.g., a lot of internet marketing revolves [around] fabricating testimonials for supplements that do very little and people who are invested in therapies inevitably tend to overrate their efficacy)."[20]

Quality manufacturers

(Note: Because the corporate purchasing of small independent producers is ongoing, this list is accurate only on the date of compilation. Despite my bias against large corporate ownership, such ownership does not necessarily mean cutting corners, and there are reputable brands still.)

Advanced Research	Apex Energetics	Bio-Tech Pharmacal
Biotics	Bluebonnet Nutrition	BodyBio PC
Boron (homeopathic)	Complementary Prescriptions	Designs for Health
Eidon Ionic Minerals	Empirical Labs	Endurance Products Company
First Line Pharmacy	Intensive Nutrition	Jarrow Formulas
Life Extension	Living Vibrant	Livon Labs
Loomis Enzymes Formulations	Mercola.com	
Metabolic Maintenance	Natural Pharm Source	Nature's Answer
Neuroscience	New Beginnings Nutritionals	Now Foods
NuMedica	Nutrient Carriers	Nutritional Frontiers
Ortho Molecular	Premier Research Labs	Protocol for Life Balance
Pure Formulas	Quicksilver Scientific	Rosita Cod Liver Oil Green Pastures Cod Liver Oil
Seeking Health	Standard Process	Thorne Research
Twin Labs	Vital Nutrients	Wellness Resources

When I feel something coming on, I immediately make a selection from my medical reservoir and the assault invariably passes. It is rare for me to deal with a cold or flu, which I attribute to living in harmony with nature. These are some of my first-line defense items. I may not use all of them and they change from time to time as I come across new information.

Echinacea	Colloidal silver
Fermented Garlic and Honey	Garlic caps
Grapefruit seed extract	Oscillococcinum
Himalayan salt	Nebulized hydrogen peroxide
Oil of oregano	Oregacillin
Olive leaf extract	Pau D'Arco Tincture
Saline nasal irrigation (neti pot)	Tea tree oil
Vitamin C	DMSO

Low carb, high fat eating

While many people enter this regimen to lose weight, a better motivation is to optimize health. (Caveat: low carb is not meant for long-term. See https://takecontrol.substack.com/p/consequences-of-low-carb-diets?utm_source=publication-search.) I began eating this way when my medical advisor, after testing, told me that while I am not insulin resistant, I was heading in that direction. I was dumbfounded. After all, I ate a multitude of whole grains and fruits—which I now know are carbohydrate-rich and convert to sugar in our bodies. This places an incessant demand on insulin production to deal with the never-ending sugar overload. This in time leads to insulin resistance and eventually diabetes as the pancreas finally says, *I'm exhausted; I can't keep up; give me a break.*

I felt better with the new regimen. And as an added benefit, the 10 pounds I had wanted to lose for several years came off in a couple of months. Here's a summary of how this regimen works:

> The idea that weight gain is simply a matter of "calories in" versus "calories out" is just plain wrong….The real weight-gain culprit is carbs in your diet.
>
> Overeating carbohydrate-rich foods can prevent a higher percentage of fats from being used for energy, and lead to an increase in fat-driven weight gain. It also raises your insulin levels, which can cause insulin resistance, followed by diabetes and a host of other chronic diseases.
>
> When you eat large amounts of sugar, fructose, bread, pasta, and any other grain products, you're essentially sending a hormonal message, via insulin, to your body that says both "keep eating" and "store more fat."
>
> When you cut carbs from sugar, fructose and grains, you need to replace those calories with healthy fats such as those from raw nuts, grass-fed butter and meats, coconut oil, egg and avocados.[21]

I no longer eat very low-carb; it did its work. Currently, what I eat is divided equally among protein, carbohydrates, and fat.

Chelation therapy

I hurt my back when I was carrying buckets of sand to fill in a low spot on my lawn. I really did a number on it and it failed to get better on its own. In fact, it got worse and worse until I experienced the greatest pain of my life. X-rays showed that I had a herniated disc.

I researched it, as I do everything, and learned that a disk often heals given enough time. However, after two months I could no longer take the pain so I scheduled surgery (desperation often leads to poor decisions). But they discovered an issue with my heart so the operation was aborted, which turned out to be a good thing—a very good thing.

As I recounted earlier, my holistic physician referred me to a naturopath position who did chelation. I hobbled in on a walker and had a consultation. She recommended and explained chelation and its coordinate, CheZone therapy. The first session was only vitamins and minerals and the next day I felt an improvement. Great beginning! And I felt better the day after each weekly session. When I arrived for my fourth session I no longer had my walker. Wow! And no more pain after the sixth. My doctor customized a regimen of vitamins and minerals to continue the healing. It's been several years now and I am back to normal, thank God.

The therapy also treated the heart issue which had prevented the back surgery.

This is the definition from the pioneer of this therapy, Dr. Frank Shallenberger.[22]

> Chelation Therapy is an intravenous treatment using a solution containing minerals, vitamins, and a special amino acid called EDTA. It is a highly effective therapy used to treat angina, coronary artery disease, atherosclerosis, heavy metal toxicity, and hypertension. CheZone therapy consists of a combination of Chelation Therapy and Ozone Therapy.

Earthing

This most valuable resource is one that you have likely never heard of. As is my wont, I researched Earthing when it caught my interest.

I had found myself running on empty by early afternoon, so much so that my day was finished; just no oomph to do much. I usually began my day around 5 AM, so by the afternoon I had expended a lot of energy. Nonetheless, the exhaustion of the afternoon felt wrong and needed to be dealt with. Thus my trying Earthing; it sounded right. Sure enough, after two months my stamina improved.

Earthing removes aches and pains too. My wife, Eve, would lay the earthing pad or place an earthing patch on an ache and it more than likely left, or at least diminished. I stand or sit at my computer with my bare feet on an earthing pad. You can learn more at www.earthing.com.

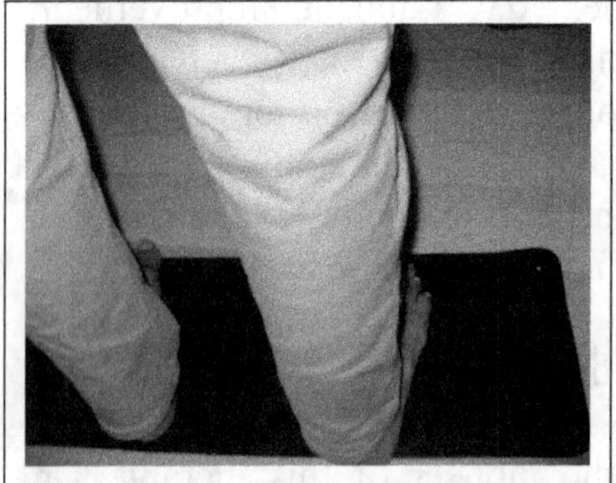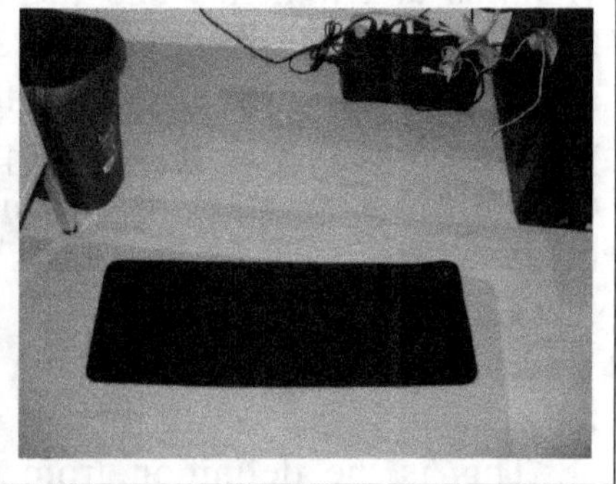

A reader commented:

I have experienced and do the things that you recommend. The only item I was not doing was Earthing. I purchased a sheet and am feeling much better. I always have had lower back aches so I thought I would give it a try. After the first night the ache went down about 50% and I feel calmer.

Acupuncture

I see my medical advisor several times a year for a tune-up. I like how he puts it: "My job is to see that you remain healthy. If you become ill, then I have failed." When I see him, I tell him of anything that's not quite right. Then he goes to work to put my energy flow in order.

I won't say more about acupuncture because most people are aware of it. But here's a photo of my alternative health practitioner at work.

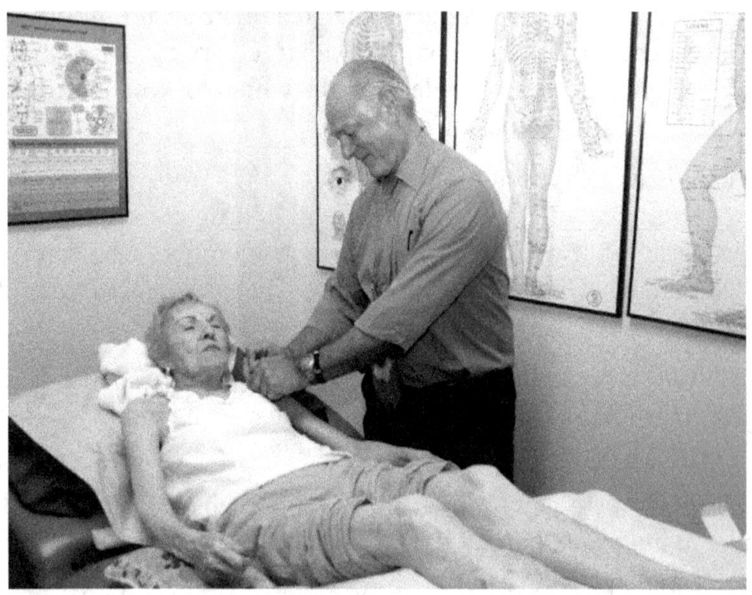

Chinese herbs

In the early 90s I developed the first and only allergy I ever had, something akin to hay fever. I went to my Chinese herbalist, who gave me an herbal remedy. She told me there is trial and error with this remedy, so let me know if it doesn't work. And it didn't. The next remedy however did the job; the allergy disappeared within a few days. Next season it returned, so I again took the remedy and once more it disappeared—but this time never to return. The way healing ought to be.

Nebulized hydrogen peroxide

The idea behind this is that heavy concentrations of microbes, such as bacteria and viruses (a.k.a. as chronic pathogen colonizations (CPC) found in periodontal disease) do oxidative damage. Good diet and antioxidant therapy will resolve the damage and cure the condition—*unless* there is an ongoing assault of pathogens. Pathogens that result in the greatest havoc are generally found in the sinuses, nose, mouth and throat, airways, and esophagus (aerodigestive tract). Chronic disease originates from this cesspool of pathogens that result in a chronic immune response, and from this comes oxidative stress. This ongoing source of damage must be dealt with, which is where nebulized hydrogen peroxide comes in.

You can listen to a discussion at https://mercola.libsyn.com/nebulized-hydrogen-peroxide-discussion-between-dr-thomas-levy-dr-mercola. Or search for "Nebulized Hydrogen Peroxide - Discussion Between Dr. Thomas Levy & Dr. Mercola."

A free e-book from Doctor Thomas Levy spells it out, *Rapid Virus Recovery*. You can download it at https://rvr.medfoxpub.com/.

This is a review on Amazon about the effectiveness of nebulized hydrogen peroxide:

Life changing! The information in this book is incredible! My whole family has had serious problems with inflammation, digestion, food sensitivities, chronic viral and bacterial infections, brain fatigue, and even illnesses from black mold poisoning.

For years we went to great doctors, took good supplements, and ate superclean—everything we were supposed to do. The improvements were happening, but very slowly and at great effort and expense. But after trying Dr. Levy's recommendations with the nebulizer, we experienced rapid, major healing and made progress in just a few days that had been taking years and thousands of our dollars to accomplish before. It is even healing the black mold illness which has been hanging over us for years.

I can't recommend this book enough. I have not felt this healthy and strong in decades and I am still amazed that something so natural, inexpensive, safe, and easy can be more effective and more powerful than anything else we've tried. Esther Vanheukelem

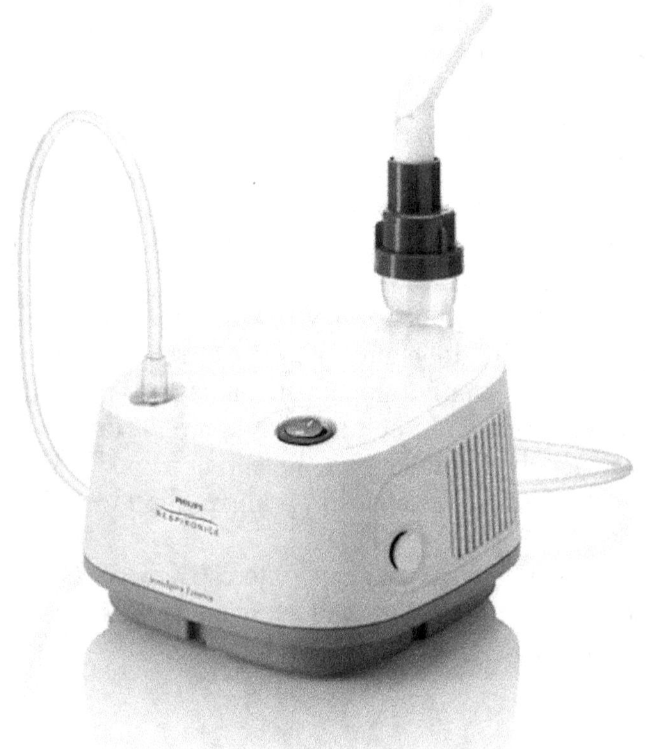

What I am using

Respironics InnoSpire Essence

Hormones

It's amazing the effect that optimized hormones have on wellness. As I wrote to someone long ago, "I've been seeing an expert on this and the improvement in my well-being is significant." They need to be bio-identical hormones by the way, not synthetic, which are the ones that have the bad rap and cause problems.

As an example of the benefit, Eve had been getting a painful quarterly cortisone injection in her thumb joint to alleviate the effect of arthritis. An unexpected benefit of optimizing her hormones was that the pain left, she regained full use of her thumb, and continued knitting. I learned that in regard to arthritis "the standard treatment is anti-inflammatory drugs, but though they often work well, all too often they provide little or no relief. Even in the best case, the drugs are intended to relieve the pain of the condition but do nothing to repair the damage or prevent the pain. Hormonal treatments, on the other hand, are 70 to 90% effective, including reversing harm done in preventing pain."[23]

You will need a specialist to optimize hormones. Don't try it on your own.

Here are two books if you have interest: Thierry Hertoghe, *The Hormone Solution* and Suzanne Somers, *Breakthrough: Eight Steps to Wellness*.

Posture

Our culture affects our health. A lifetime of messaging of how we should look eventually erases our memory of living in harmony with how we are designed. For example, high heels work against body mechanics and result in the chest and lower back pushed forward causing pressure on the knees and the balls of the feet, which results in various medical conditions. The same applies to furniture that works against the natural design of our bodies. Chronic pain and poor health result. Most people no longer know what good health and fitness are. They have forgotten how to inhabit their bodies as nature intended.

Everything you do is affected by posture; it is foundational to good health. I learned this method: www.GokhaleMethod.com.

The Gokhale Method uses primal posture and movement to help you re-establish your body's structural integrity and regain a pain-free life.

I have had to deal with a weakened back since my early 20's when I foolishly carried the front-end of a window air conditioner up a flight of stairs. It seemed every few years it would flare up, and it had recently done so when I came across this concept of posture's effect on our wellbeing. So after my initial review of the website, I carefully studied Esther Gokhale's book and changed my posture: how I walk, sit, stand, and sleep. I also took her posture class. I now feel a strength and well-being in how I carry myself, and have had no back pain since I successfully dealt with a herniated disc in 2017 (which I wrote about earlier).

A woman who read my book offered her experience.

Correct posture is very important as we age. I do spinal exercises; the CD I use is called Aging Backwards (www.essentrics.com) with Miranda Esmone-White. I continue to do these exercises about four times a week, and I measure one inch taller than when I started!

In summary, I consider the seemingly inevitable worn-out parts, degeneration, and dysfunction to be reversible. We can and should expect to function well into our higher decades, even to our end of days.

CBD Oil and Cannabis

I researched this primarily for my wife and asked my holistic physician about it. His patients use cannabis with good results. Regarding CBD oil, he recommended Quicksilver nanoemulsified Colorado Hemp oil. It's important to get a reputable brand; they are not all equal.

The CBD oil helped reduce the effects of Eve's stress as well as aches and pains. I decided to try it as well because it has so much going for it. I did not see anything in particular change, but then again I did not have specific issues to deal with. Eve subsequently graduated to medical marijuana because the THC component adds to the efficacy of CBD oil alone. It was worth it for her.

Here are several ailments cannabis deals with (and there are many more):

- Arthritis, osteoarthritis or rheumatoid arthritis
- Degenerative neurological disorders such as dystonia
- Multiple sclerosis
- Parkinson's disease
- Post-traumatic stress disorder (PTSD)
- Epilepsy and seizures

It is best to begin a relationship with a medical professional that specializes in cannabis. There is so much research being done that a general practitioner does not have the time to stay on top of it in my opinion.

Low Dose Naltrexone (LDN)

My health practitioner recommended LDN to deal with the chronic inflammation and immune system damage from long undetected gluten intolerance. It strengthened my immune system and does a host of other things as well.

It triggers endorphin production, which helps boost immune function, and has anti-inflammatory effects on the central nervous system. Doctor Joseph Mercola

Here are some user comments:

It is like a miracle, healing the gut lining, helping the intestines to absorb nutrients again, and keeps the immune system from going down due to dairy and gluten.

3 mg or 4.5 mg of LDN is taken before a person goes to bed. It feels like taking a vitamin, has no side effects, is cheap, works fantastic, and is amazing.

It blocks the opiate receptor sites that dairy/gluten stimulate, that cause the immune system go down. LDN lets the immune system work properly. LDN heals the stomach/intestines, helps stop hair loss, helps the immune system, helps depression, gives energy, helps mood, helps stop cravings, helps personality, helps the liver to remove heavy metals, and helps every cell of the body, etc. Wow! It is like a miracle!

I had taken it for three years or so. My immune system and inflammation have since healed. I cannot say definitively that it was the LDN that did it because of other things I was doing to deal with the problem. I have considered using it again preventatively, but I am doing enough to maintain my health that I do not feel it is needed.

- Learn more at https://www.ldnresearchtrust.org/ and www.LowDoseNaltrexone.org.
- This is a video by doctor about it: https://www.youtube.com/watch?v=2sYAxH24kuQ. I suggest you also read the comments from users that benefited from it.

Alternative care as a financial investment

Many are deterred from using alternative health practitioners and products because insurance covers few of them. You pay it all, although lab tests ordered by a physician are generally covered by insurance.

From my experience, it's first necessary to understand and believe your health and well-being will substantially improve to justify the cost. It begins as a faith effort until you *know* the truth of the matter. At the beginning of this journey you must swim upstream against the mindset of the general population and the vast majority of institutions. The primary driver is the determined obstructionism to alternative medical care by the Conventional Medical Complex.

I have found that it costs less over time to pay out of pocket compared to insurance paid conventional disease management (not prevention and optimal health). How is this so? Foremost, you avoid a diseased body and becoming a ward of the medical system. What is feeling well worth?

Second, because you remain healthy you avoid illness and the often-considerable expense associated with it, even with insurance. For example, my brother spent one night in the hospital and left with an $1100 bill—and that's with Medicare and supplemental health insurance. That would have paid for a lot of alternative healthcare. And what about lost wages and productivity from ill health you avoid?

But when it's all said and done, improved health and quality of life justify the expense, learning, and effort to become confident in making your own medical decisions.

My health regimen

As the particulars of well-being are unique to me, so are they for you. I lay out my current regimen so you have an idea of what it takes to not only feel well but also to thrive when so much around us is toxic.

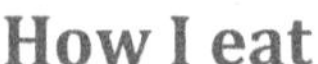

How I eat

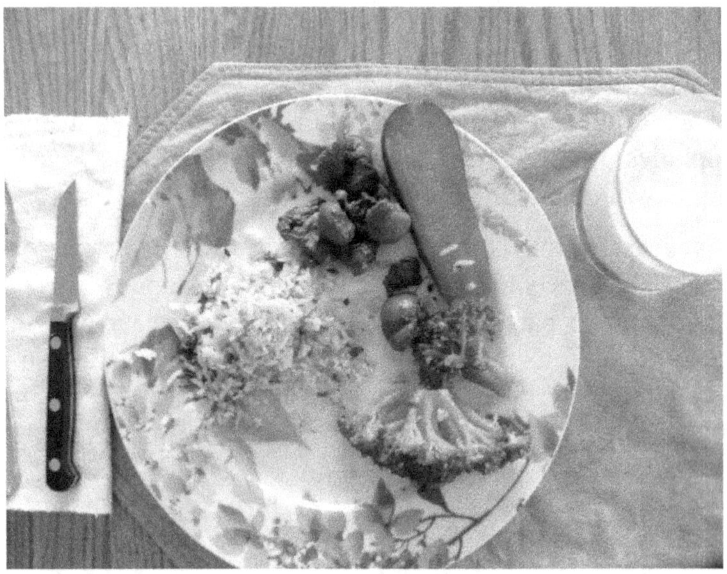

Although what I eat at lunch of course varies, this meal is not untypical: Rice with seaweed, broccoli, kidney, fermented pickle and kefir.

The foods I choose are almost entirely organic or equivalent. I don't care to eat out because not only is it rare to find organically sourced foods but also foodborne illness is a risk. And I've come to enjoy cooking; it's a creative and wholesome activity. Nonetheless, I do not forgo social gathering around food. Because I live healthy, my body is able to deal with any suboptimal food and contamination.

I buy my meats and vegetables almost entirely from local farmers who I know and whose practices are biologically sound. Same with dairy products that I buy from a farm store who sources them from suppliers with integrity. I do buy vegetables from time to time at the supermarket, but almost always organic. Even then, the profit motive rules most corporations, so while they produce USDA organically labeled foods in quantities for the mass-market, they use loopholes in the organic standards to increase yield and reduce cost. Their sophisticated marketing is intended to deceive the consumer into thinking it's the same as the local farmer whose practices and integrity you know, in which case it need not be organic.

Here is a comment from a woman who understands how USDA organic standards cannot be relied on:

> Chances are that people who think they are buying totally organic food in the supermarket only have a 50/50 chance of actually eating organically. There are so many loopholes in the laws and so much corruption. Some people will do anything for money.

I have been gluten-free for years because I had been gluten intolerant. The concentration of gluten in today's grains is so much more than in the past and it harms many people unknowingly. Here's a video from this person who writes: "Going gluten-free was a random experiment that ended up changing my life for the better. My mental health and quality of life have improved dramatically."
https://www.youtube.com/watch?v=ckWbgz9Hesk. You will find more detail in this article by Doctor Thomas Levy: *Medical warning: Gluten allergies affect everyone*
https://www.peakenergy.com/articles/nh20190930/Medical-warning:-Gluten-allergies-affect-everyone/. You may wish to experiment and avoid gluten *totally* to see if nagging problems leave. It has happened for many.

I generally eat between 7 AM and 5 PM. The energy that would otherwise be used for digestion is now available during the night to power the body's maintenance activities. I've stop snacking, and if I feel hungry between meals, I'll have a cup of coffee with a dollop of ghee or some kombucha. But I'm flexible and listen to my body should I need something more substantial.

Fortunately, I grew up in a household that did not have much use for sugar. My alternative medical practitioner told me, "If there were one thing to recommend to my patients, it would be to substantially reduce sugar."

Lastly, I change how I eat from time to time as new information comes my way. Makes life interesting as well.

Probiotics sourced from fermented foods

I stopped probiotics supplements when I learned that cultured foods have a vastly greater diversity and quantity of probiotic strains. And we're talking foods, not pills—a nice change. They are tasty as well. Some of the foods I ferment are pickles, sauerkraut, kefir, kombucha, yogurt, vegetables, and kimchee. By the way, don't throw out the juices; they're a great store of probiotics. I drink them straight, use them to ferment vegetables, add a couple of tablespoons to soak grains overnight; there are recipes for their use.

Be sure to avoid the additive and sugar-laden brands of probiotic foods (they are the ones not refrigerated). Also, you hear all the time that yogurt is a good source of probiotics, but because the milk is pasteurized, which destroys bacteria, probiotic strains must be added back in, which is a pittance of what was there naturally.

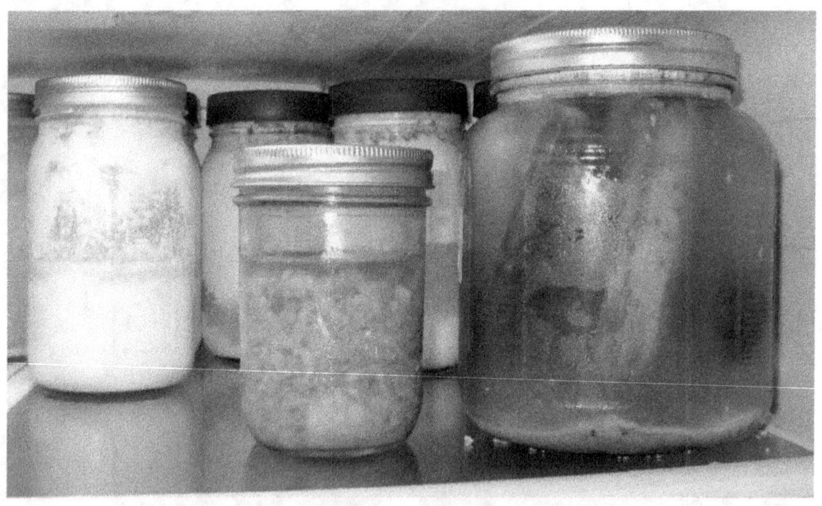

Left to right: kefir, sauerkraut, pickles; not shown is yogurt, salad dressing, kombucha, and kimchi

This is where I learned to culture food. The link is to stories of remarkable recovery. https://www.culturedfoodlife.com/lives-touched

Supplements

I am not taking supplements currently because I intuitively feel complete with my nutrient dense diet, and I haven't discerned deficiencies or had recent testing done. When I feel the need, I test my vitamin and mineral levels in consultation with my alternative health advisor to determine if I need to supplement and what they should be.

Below I include some of the reasons I have taken various supplements to illustrate the importance of actually knowing what a supplement will do for you and not because it merely sounds good and "it can't hurt" (it can).

- Coenzyme Q10 (coQ10)—Ubiquinol is preferred. As an antioxidant it spares others antioxidants from being used up and supports others.

- Essential Fatty Acids (in place of fish oil supplements)—I use Parent Essential Oils (https://www.yes-supplements.com/products/yes-ultimate-efas.html) because direct omega three supplementation has dangers associated with it. My doctor, to whom I introduced it, was impressed with this product. You can read about it in Brian Peskin's book, PEO Solution - Conquering Cancer, Diabetes and Heart Disease with Parent Essential Oils. It's a great read!

- Magnesium—I began this supplement to deal with the cellular health of my heart. But it does a host of other things as well. From Jon Barron's website: "Magnesium is the activating mineral for close to 400 different enzyme reactions in the body (that we know about)—more than any other mineral. Too little magnesium literally impacts your body negatively in hundreds of ways." https://www.jonbarron.org/herbal-library/nutraceuticals/magnesium

- Vitamin C —A superb antioxidant; I used to combine 1 teaspoon with ½ teaspoon baking soda each morning.

- Digestive enzymes—I would take before my main meal to supplement the enzymes that have declined with age.

- Vitamin B complex—It does more than I can say here, so be sure it's measured in your nutritional labs.
- Vitamin D—I used to take 5000 units daily, but I have recently discovered that vitamin D from sunlight has dozens of metabolites that that act like stem cells in that they can accomplish whatever is needed. This is in contrast to vitamin D3 supplementation which has only one pathway from the liver. And there is more to it that you can see here:

  https://www.youtube.com/watch?v=eg0PBu79QqY
- E Tocotrienols—Antioxidant and plaque stabilizer among other things.
- Vitamin K—In dealing with vascular calcification (a heart issue), K2 removes calcium. From a doctor, "People getting a lot of K2 from their diet have less cardiovascular disease later in life. We get K2 from animals that eat grass…."

The exercises I do

As with everything else in my health regimen, this changes from time to time according to the needs of my body and new information.

- Walk 1 ¼ miles daily at a good rate
- Mostly hand weights two or three times a week depending on the season and what else I'm doing.
- Swim most days; not so much in the cold weather although that may change.

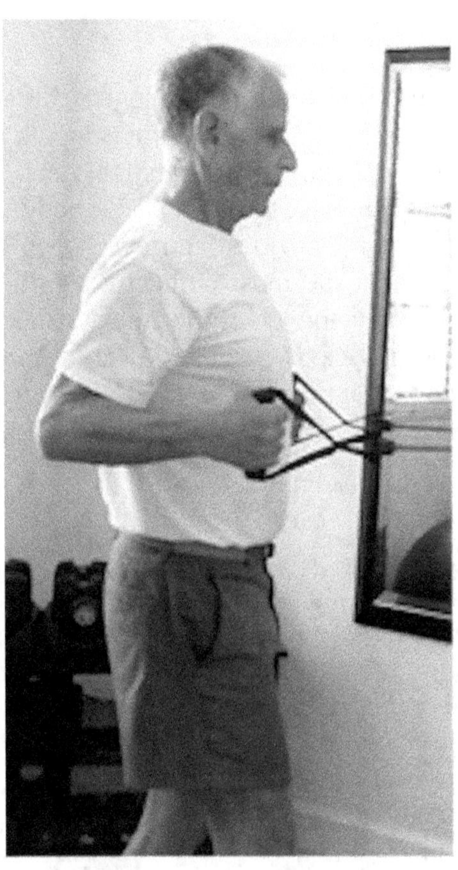

Teeth

It is crucial to have good teeth. Our health determines the condition of our gums and teeth. It's a shame how many people have decayed and missing teeth and suffer grievous oral problems.

Dr. [Weston] Price noticed an incredible increase in tooth decay when people began eating processed foods. When he began his journey around the world, he found native people who were still eating their traditional diets had nearly perfect teeth.[24]

Our teeth not only reflect the condition of our health but also contribute to illness and disease.

The bulk of CPC (chronic pathogen colonization) in the body is located in the sinuses, nose, mouth and throat, airways, and esophagus (aerodigestive tract). Although CPC infections can exist throughout the body in the cells lining hollow organs, cavities, and even open spaces, the CPCs that result in the most clinically significant health issues are generally found on the mucosal and epithelial surfaces of the oral cavity, sinuses, pharyngeal areas, and the lungs. CPC continually assaults the gut with new pathogen and toxin exposures with every swallow.[25]

When my dentist advised me to floss many years ago, I did so out of principle and was not happy to add this to my morning regimen. But soon enough it became a habit and just part of living. (Isn't it wonderful how you can reprogram yourself?) My hygienist saw that my gums showed damage from toothpicks. She told me that toothpicks can be harmful and suggested using an interdental brush; these are the ones I use: https://www.gumbrand.com/dental-picks-advanced.html.

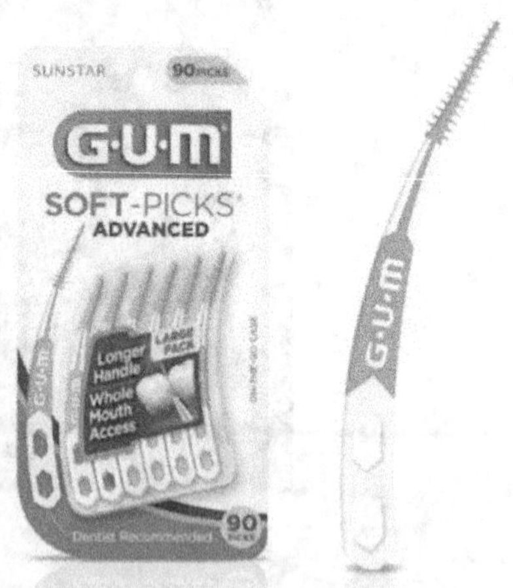

My hygienist saw that with all my effort that a small area of my gums showed a slight softness. She suggested a salt and baking soda mix (50-50) for short-term use. Three weeks later she said the difference was dramatic; and it diminished staining. I now add water to baking soda to make a slurry into which I dip the interdental brush. I also use a water flosser.

The result of all this? As the child exclaimed in the 1950s ad, "Look Ma, no cavities!

How I care for my teeth

- I brush *whenever* I eat something; I don't like continuing to taste what I ate.
- I use a non-EMF red light therapy electric toothbrush (Bristl 21 https://bristlscience.com) as well as a standard one.
- I use an interdental brush after eating.
- I floss after my last meal and use a water flosser. This is the order.
- I see my dental hygienist twice a year for cleaning. And now that I'm older it's become three times, for it's not only for cleaning but also a safeguard should something be developing that needs attention.

Biological dentistry

I experienced pain on a particular tooth and went to my conventional dentist to check it out. (I would have used a biological dentist but there were none local.) She said after questioning and an x-ray, "The nerve is dying and you need to get a root canal: quicker the better." I read something about root canals that wasn't good, and recalled an interview of a biological dentist I had seen, and so began my research. Well, what an eye-opener about the dangers of root canals and much more.

I discovered a biological dentist about an hour and a quarter from me, longer than I would like, but began working with this wonderful husband and wife team. No need for a root canal and other potential issues for dealt with.

Here are resources about biological dentistry:

This is the interview from which I learned about biological dentistry: https://takecontrol.substack.com/p/carlo-litano-biological-dentistry.

I found this documentary on root canals educational. I did not care for the dramatizations but the dentists who spoke were top notch: https://rumble.com/v23dr46-special-presentation-root-cause-documentary.html

This is an excellent introduction to biological dentistry: *Chew on this...: but don't swallow* by Dr. Blanche Grube. https://store.bookbaby.com/book/chew-on-this1

This is an extensive explanation from Swiss Biohealth (www.swiss-biohealth.com): https://sds.directus.app/assets/5f95a9f9-b7a3-4c90-bb55-96dac90bbc57/THE-SWISS-BIOHEALTH-CONCEPT.pdf

You can learn more and search for a biological dentist at these organizations:

The International Academy of Oral Medicine and Toxicology (IAOMT)
International Academy of Biological Dentistry & Medicine (IABDM)
Holistic Dental Association
Consumers for Dental Choice
International Association of Mercury Safe Dentists
Talk International

Institutionalized Medicine

Sad to say, most people expect their older years to be a saga of chronic disease and diminished capacity. They experience the quality of their lives deteriorate as ill-health increasingly consumes their time, focus, and money—not to mention how depleting it is to family and caregivers.

We have relinquished the control of our bodies to the medical system. We go to the doctor by default rather than think through the problem and how best to deal with it, how it has been done in harmony with nature for thousands of years. More doctoring is not better, especially considering the abysmal results in people's health that have resulted in the last 100 or so years of conditioning us to abdicate common sense in favor of medical orthodoxy—if we don't approve, it's wrong.

Western medicine focuses on treating disease, the *symptoms* of ill health, not the promotion of wellness and thus the avoidance of disease.

> The Western model is mechanistic whereas other, more ancient medical models are holistic, focusing on treating the entire body. Western medicine…is focused on treating a specific health problem, often by the application of physical treatments. In fact, this led to an emphasis on treating symptoms rather than underlying causes.[26]

The conventional disease management (not health optimization) industry (what I term the Conventional Medical Complex) consists of:

- pharmaceutical companies (Big Pharma).
- the medical establishment (medical societies, schools, scientists, hospitals, and doctors).
- industrial agriculture.
- large food manufacturers.
- insurance companies.
- government (politicians with conflicts of interest and agencies beholden to industry, such as the Federal Drug Administration (FDA) and the Centers for Disease Control (CDC).
- mass media which masks the deceit, error, and harm of the Medical Complex while promoting its agenda. Over time its

messaging becomes embedded in our collective consciousness as unchallengeable orthodoxy.

Why doctors are not always the trusted resource we believe

Most doctors…have the capacity to understand
the truth but they don't pursue it.
(Dr. Joseph Mercola)

Doctors you know and trust may mean well, but they often unwittingly spread misinformation and offer poor advice.

Doctors, while well-intentioned, have by and large become untrustworthy for the simple fact that they stopped thinking for themselves and fell into a corporate for-profit scheme that depends on chronic illness. Few are those who buck the system, do their own research rather than getting their information from pharmaceutical reps, and focus on patient education about preventive strategies that don't involve costly drugs or surgical interventions.[27]

Here is a post from a reader at www.mercola.com:

I know a very honest and respected doctor who does not understand why some people do not follow their doctors' advice. Well, because as wonderful as you are, you are not the person doing the research. You are depending on someone else's research who may or may not be ethical.

Here's an example of misinformation aimed at doctors to increase opioid sales.

The massive increase in opioid sales and subsequent addiction rates have been traced back to an orchestrated marketing plan aimed at misinforming doctors about the drug's addictive potential, and it is this false advertising campaign that seeded the current opioid epidemic.[28]

In addition to its disinformation campaigns, the pharmaceutical industry works hard at discrediting holistic, naturopathic, and natural health practitioners. It scares them that people might recognize that drugs only mask symptoms *and create more of them*, and they don't cure anything.

It takes courage to speak truth to power in the medical cartel. It is costly to publicly object to a dangerous product or practice when industry owns the media and maintains kennels of conflicted staff-scientists and ravening lawfare wolves.

If perchance a licensed doctor wanted to use therapeutic measures not on the government approved standard practice list he would face professional censure, insurance complications and criminal prosecution. Physicians are hobbled by a system that enables pharmaceutical monopoly and destroys any remnant of health freedom. After decades of grueling medical education, few are willing to cast their professional and economic fate to the fickle winds of legal entanglement. Fortunately a hand-full of doctors are confident enough to ignore rules and may save us all.[29]

This is the experience of a woman who did her research, made her own decisions on cancer treatment, and recovered despite standard care guidelines.

As for slash-poison-burn therapies [surgery-chemotherapy-radiation], what one doctor admitted to me behind a closed door after I made a dramatic recovery was, "What we do does not work." He was curious but afraid to ask, "How did you do it?" because, by having an open mind, it would negate his years of training and place him in the perilous position of needing to consider offering his patients "nonstandard treatment" which means he could lose his license.

I realized that, if forced to choose, many doctors would choose to see me dead rather than jeopardize the license they had worked so hard to obtain. So, the moral of the story is you need to be in control of all decision-making, educate yourself and act in your own best interest.

Doctors are trained in drug therapy. Alternative solutions do not fit the standards of care mandated by the pharmaceutical model, insurance companies, and medical authorities. Doctors rarely consider alternate healthcare, and when they do, they fear being censured or losing their license.

The pharmaceutical model, which substitutes chemistry for herbology, is often propped up by dubious scientific evidence and a broad (and biased) regulatory structure that makes it difficult for even age-old alternative treatments to advance.[30]

Insurance companies restrict how doctors can practice, reimbursing only for "proven" remedies. They will not pay for most alternative health solutions because they lack the expensive research needed to obtain government approval. They disregard the history of successful use, copious anecdotal evidence, and credible research that is available.

Do insurance companies have the well-being of their policyholders as a priority? As recounted below, they are not always ethical. A doctor related this story:

> I have a friend who is an acupuncturist now and he told me a story that he witnessed an adjuster pick up a two-foot stack of claims forms, walk them over to the rubbish basket and drop them in. Half of those people will never follow up, so the insurance company saves money on paying claims. The insurance game is "delay, delay, delay, deny."

Most doctors are ignorant of nutritional healing and the effect that food has on health.

> The virtual epidemic of diabetes that has swept the West and especially the US is no doubt in part due to the ingredients and additives in many foods. It is difficult to find food in the US that has no additives or chemicals of any sort, especially Big Food grown, packaged and shipped from agricultural corporations.[31]

Doctors often convey pessimism to their patients, directly or unwittingly, and the mind-body connection works in reverse to worsen illness.

> Too many doctors are deeply pessimistic about the possibility of people getting better, and they communicate their pessimism to patients and families. Many of the patients who come to see me have been told by doctors, in one way or another, that they will not get better, that they will have to learn to live with their problems or expect to

die from them, that medicine has nothing more to offer them.[32]

The Conventional Medical Complex

The entrenched medical establishment is often characterized by corporate greed, government corruption, fear of change, and indifference. It generally opposes alternative care because it offers competition, which translates into reduced profits, status, power, and job security.

> It is difficult to get a man to understand something when his salary depends on him not understanding it. (Upton Sinclair)

The highly respected integrative medical researcher and practitioner Dr. Andrew Weil says,

> There are many vested interests that are making out from the present system and they will be very resistant to change, but the whole system is going down so at some point that will all have to change.[33]

More than just the loss of income, if too many actually improve their health, many in conventional medicine would lose their jobs. This fact cannot be ignored, and it is a significant reason why conventional medicine drags its feet when it comes to recommending and implementing the use of alternative solutions.

Here's an example of the reaction from a scientist and a doctor when a new health technology was presented. (This is from Clint Ober's book, *Grounding*, a fascinating technology I use. I provide a brief overview in the section, *Alternative Health Solutions*.)

> Most scientists or doctors had no desire to get involved or lend their name to anything out of left field like this, something with no scientific history or legitimacy. One scientist…said he wouldn't believe it even if it were published in the *New England Journal of Medicine*. One doctor told me that even if what I was saying were true, why would he tell patients to take off their shoes and *get well for free*?[34] [emphasis mine]

It difficult for doctors to reach a view contrary to the consensus. However, all too often things that were once considered safe and accepted were later found to be harmful, although an alternative view of the danger was available.

It was only a few years ago that four out of five doctors were known to have recommended a certain brand of cigarettes. Fifty years ago doctors puffed away and found nothing wrong with their patients doing the same.

Of course, a few activists warned against the dangers of cigarette smoking, but the doctors had their say, dismissing such claims because they never learned in medical school that cigarette smoking was dangerous. There was no opposite viewpoint for physicians to consider, so their minds were made up by clever marketing.[35]

Nevertheless, there are doctors who go where truth leads. An alternative health physician wrote this to me:

I would like to honor the knowledge that I received in medical school. Deficient as it was in conveying the concept of the unity of body, mind, and spirit, the knowledge acquired at med school was incredible, true, and accurate. The failing was in integrating not only other modalities, such as acupuncture and homeopathy but also the different organ systems in the body. The endocrine system, immune system, neurological system, etc. are studied separately, and if there is a problem from outside the field of the specialist, the patient is referred to the "appropriate" specialist.

Additionally, I have met many MDs who practice more holistically, who I greatly respect in stepping outside of their comfortable boundaries.

Should a member of the Conventional Medical Complex recognize the dangers imposed upon the public and be bold about such insight, he will lose status and prestige among his peers, not to mention his financial well-being. The doctor who recognizes the truth of the matter faces a great decision: will he have the courage to follow wherever truth leads? Being a trailblazer may entail grave consequences to one's lifestyle, but oh the soul growth that ensues!

As consumers of medical care it's imperative that we think for ourselves, that we embrace original and unfettered thinking that has escaped blinding tradition and narrow convention. It requires concerted effort to escape the gravity of the conventional healthcare mindset and its propaganda. We need to seek alternative sources of information and courageously act on what resonates with us and we recognize to be true.

Notwithstanding all that I have said, conventional medicine provides a counterbalance to unbridled zealous efforts to precipitously replace the old with the new. Healthcare, like everything else in civilization, does best by evolution, not revolution. But a steep price is paid, that of retarding real progress. However, over time that which is true prevails.

False science and corporate disinformation

The Medical Complex has systematized the falsification of the scientific method to avoid public awareness and government action about research that would harm its profits. These are their methods as outlined by the Union of Concerned Scientists:[36]

3. The Fake—Conduct counterfeit science and try to pass it off as legitimate research.
4. The Blitz—Harass scientists who speak out with results or views inconvenient for industry.
5. The Diversion—Manufacture uncertainty about science where little or none exists.
6. The Screen—Buy credibility through alliances with academia or professional societies.
7. The Fix—Manipulate government officials or processes to influence policy inappropriately.

Royal Lee, founder of Standard Process, whole food-based nutritional supplements (www.standardprocess.com), wrote this about vitamins in reference to so called experts. "The question arises: Are synthetic imitations equal to the genuine, which cost far more? Many so-called "experts" say that there is no difference. Notoriously, experts can usually be found to express any opinion commercial interests need to promote their wares or keep people out of jail. Here is a case for everyone to carefully examine the facts for themselves."[37]

I've gone on long enough; you get the idea.

BODY, MIND, SPIRIT CONNECTION

The spiritual component of health

This book has primarily been about physical poisons that harm our material bodies. But equally important, because we are triune or threefold beings, are the spiritual poisons that harm our souls and the mental poisons that damage our minds, for they affect our physical bodies as surely as day follows night.

It is difficult for most people to comprehend the spiritual aspect of dis-ease. This is how I see it work: disease is integral to personal evolution and spiritual growth. It is an attention-getter and often a wake-up call to attend to those areas of mind, body, and spirit that are that are disrupted, not in harmony with the cosmos.

The condition of your body has an enormous effect on your psyche. It requires vision, commitment, and effort to trust your inner compass and the messages of your body to heal and stay well rather than rely on medical authority. A superior physical nature lends itself to achieving spiritual potential.

I know many spiritually minded men and women who are hard after truth. They diligently seek to live in time the values of eternity. They are valiant to do right, to be loyal cosmic citizens of high ethical conduct and moral conscience. But all too often their quest for truth fails to extend to their physical bodies.

> Ram Dass [a well-known spiritual teacher], 71, suffered a massive stroke seven years ago that resulted in long stays in the hospital and nursing home....(He) admitted that while he paid attention to his spiritual side, he often ignored his physical health. "I did not care for my body," he said. "I cared for my psychology and my soul, but I never cared for my body.[38]

The physical wellbeing of these spiritually minded men and women is not as different as it might be from the population at large who suffer from poor health and chronic disease. I attribute this to a bias towards spiritual unity. It is spiritual growth that is important; give as little attention to the body as possible because it takes away from spiritual focus and mind mastery. As a result, spiritually minded folk tend to contemn the physical as inferior to the spiritual. They are not! They are decidedly equal when you consider their origin before the I AM differentiated them. The spiritual and material are two facets the Infinite. This extends to all things material, including our bodies. You cannot have one without the other. For example, you cannot have a healthy population when the planet is sick. Neither can you actualize your spiritual potential when your body is not well.

Over the years I've read how a particular solution didn't work for someone or even caused an adverse reaction. Those of us who have been serious about holistic healing know that each of us being unique, solutions that work for one may not be suitable for another. What is the solution to this quandary of what solutions to apply to yourself?

Modern culture places great emphasis on logical intelligence and evidence-based thinking in decision making. But clearly, it doesn't always work with alternative medicine. Personal decisions must also include the intuitive side of our being, inner knowing, heart discernment. The still-small-voice is all too often ignored when it speaks, *This is the way, walk in it.*

The effect of health on spiritual guidance

While this book is primarily about achieving bodily health, it is important to know its effect upon the other two domains of our makeup, mind and spirit. An unhealthy body hinders the spiritual life.

> The Adjuster [indwelling Spirit] remains with you in all disaster and through every sickness which does not wholly destroy the mentality. But how unkind knowingly to defile or otherwise deliberately to pollute the physical body, which must serve as the earthly tabernacle of this marvelous gift from God. All physical poisons greatly retard the efforts of the Adjuster to exalt the material mind, while the mental poisons of fear, anger, envy, jealousy, suspicion, and intolerance likewise tremendously interfere with the spiritual progress of the evolving soul. (Urantia Book, 110:1.5)

To the degree that your body is healthy, strong, and responsive, your physical nature more easily responds to spirit guidance. Otherwise, the spirit and flesh remain in a never-ending struggle that results in confusion and stress.

Physical poisons not only harm the body and prevent the mind from functioning well, they greatly retard the effort of the indwelling Spirit and other celestial influences to impart spiritual insight. By contrast, physical health makes a way for its reception.

> It is to the mind of perfect poise, housed in a body of clean habits, stabilized neural energies, and balanced chemical function ... that a maximum of light and truth can be imparted.... (Urantia Book, 110:6.4)

The positive value of health is not only the negative avoidance of illness and disease. A spiritually aligned individual is not only guided to embrace physically healthy habits but also eschew "the mental poisons of fear, anger, envy, jealousy, suspicion, and intolerance."[39] Looking from the bottom up, a healthy lifestyle facilitates an upreach toward God consciousness. Looking from the top down we generally first become ill on a spiritual level. If this progresses unrecognized, then we develop symptoms on a molecular level. If still unrecognized it progresses to problems on a chemical level which can be identified by lab tests. If not handled at this point, the physical body will manifest symptoms—you get sick and become diseased.

Physical ailments lead to introspection

Don't look with dread when your body is experiencing disharmony. Rather, it is an invitation to examine yourself and incorporate mind and spirit. Here are two examples:

> I found myself stubbing my toe frequently. I didn't think much of it and continued to stub my toes every so often. Finally, it caused a toenail fungus for which I had to see a doctor.

> Fortunately, I had come to the place in my life where I didn't pass off things wrong with me as just the way life is. I looked deeper into why I had created a habit of injuring my toes in this way. And as is usually the case, because I sincerely wanted to know, the answer came to me.

> I had made it a habit to be as efficient as I could in my life. Whenever I was walking somewhere, my mind would be off thinking about something else. After all, why waste

time focusing on where I'm walking when I could be making better use of it?

I recognized such efficiency was wrong headed and realized where it came from—my childhood. My mother was a young widow was two small children. She was very anxious about money and I picked up that worry about there not being enough. Because scarcity is how the world thinks, therefore use as little as possible of everything—your energy, your time, your money— because life is against you. It's this doctrine of scarcity that really caused me not to focus on where I walked. (As an added benefit I am less likely to go from one room to another and forget why.)

I've learned that life is abundant. I now take the time needed to do things well. I now live more focused, in the moment, being here now. I am grateful that this minor hurt began a profound reflection that changed my life.

I also realized what it means to think of things as a whole (holistically), how the body, the mind, and the spirit are coordinate.

Here is the second example from a doctor skilled in intuiting the mind body connection.[40]

Adrian had come in two weeks before with a chronic, strange sort of pain in her foot. Underneath that there seemed to be some reluctance to decide which direction to move in her life—where to step next, so to speak! Though she had before given the impression of being supremely confident and well-established in her professional work, I pointed out in that session what this symptom seemed to be saying. She was taken aback. Her face registered an initial suspicious surprise, and then her voice dropped. She confided, "I have been thinking of other work. The truth is, my job is not so stable. In fact, there's talk of eliminating my position…" As she left that day, she paused, looked back at me, and said "thank you for seeing me the way I really am."

Control your end of days

The healthier you are in body, the easier in mind and spirit for the indwelling God Fragment to communicate and guide your steps into the ways of health, happiness, and true success. Your indwelling Spirit is deeply concerned with and seeks to contribute to your physical well-being. Developing a lifestyle attuned to his piloting greatly increases the chances that you will live out your days strong and vibrant—even participating in how your days will end.

> And when Jacob had made an end of commanding his sons, he gathered up his feet into the bed, and yielded up the ghost, and was gathered unto his people. (Genesis 49:33)

> Then Abraham gave up the ghost, and died in a good old age, an old man, and full of years; and was gathered to his people. (Genesis 25:8)

> And Isaac gave up the ghost, and died, and was gathered unto his people, being old and full of days. (Genesis 35:29)

> And Moses was a hundred and twenty years old when he died: his eye was not dim, nor his natural force abated. (Deuteronomy 34:7)

My initial motivation to learn about health and take control of it was the fear of disability and old-age decrepitude. I realize now there is a better reason: optimize my connection with spirit. With that in place, good health follows because of intelligent decision-making derived holistically from the three levels of our being: material, mindal, spiritual.

In this regard, most health professionals deal with physical health, and on occasion, mental clarity and emotional control; spiritual health is not comprehended and unlikely to be addressed. Therefore, because the health of the body is the material foundation of the spiritual life, each of us must provide those favorable physical conditions that support a personal relationship with the divine Spirit within and the Universal Father without.

Physical changes brought about by spiritual health

A spiritual connection makes it easier to remake energy forms in your mind. Neuroplasticity means that habits can rewire your brain, favorably or unfavorably. For example, a negative outlook on life, depression, and anxiety create mind forms that makes those conditions more likely to continue. Fortunately, the reverse is also true.

> The thoughts that we think emit a charge to the emotions, and that charge also emits a signal to the physical body.[41] Every thought wave creates a different motion in the atoms and cells of the body.[42]

> Just keep opening and not closing. Wait until you see what happens to you. You can even affect the health of your body with your energy flow. When you start to feel the tendency of an illness coming on, you just relax and open. When you open, you bring more energy into the system, and it can heal. Energy can heal, and that's why love can heal. As you explore your inner energy, a whole world of discovery opens up to you.[43]

Values such as love, compassion, mercy, forgiveness, and understanding are divine attributes of our heavenly Father. These word-forms of spirit-language come alive by spirit-energy substance. (Spirit-energy has attributes such as form, color, shape, texture, light, and vibration.) We take on spirit-energy as we incorporate its values into our lives. It is by this means that spiritual information flows into our consciousness and becomes hardwired into our physical body through the chakra system.

The spiritual nature

I have been recounting how the health of the physical body and the soundness of the mind affect the growth of the spiritual nature. I was asked this question: *What is the spiritual nature*? I answered:

> Spirit is not merely an abstract concept; it is an actual substance. A person who has developed their spiritual nature emanates energy similar to a magnet that has a force field. That's why if you are sensitive enough you can

feelingly discern the spiritual nature of a sufficiently developed soul.

How do you acquire a spiritual nature? Think of the physical-material body, how it begins as a single cell and in time evolves into a full human being. Somewhat like that single biological cell, God endows each of us at conception with an embryonic soul, the place of our spiritual nature. Our soul grows each time a moral choice between right and wrong is made, each time we choose to do the will of the heavenly Father rather than our will, each time we lovingly serve and fulfill the needs of others. It is up to us to make those choices that allow the indwelling Spirit of the heavenly Father to grow our soul and develop our spiritual nature.

Our spiritual and material natures in balance

This is worthwhile repeating: For some there is neglect of the spiritual life and a focus on the physical-material life. It is likewise dangerous to overemphasize the spiritual to the neglect of the physical. The inner spiritual life and the outer material-physical life must be balanced and in harmony to be healthy. Material substance and spirit substance are two sides of the same coin, having originally been one in the I AM. To regard the body as inferior to the spiritual, even to the slightest degree, is to disdain the material creation of the Creator. Balance and harmony are the watchwords of creation.

Rest, spirit connectivity, and communion

This is my experience: I have found that rest and relaxation are crucial to spiritual liaison, which in turn has a potent effect upon health. Such a connection enables me to think about my health from a cosmic perspective. Here's what I mean by a cosmic perspective: communing with divine Spirit who indwells me, the source of all that's good, true and beautiful. Such thinking illuminates how to live in harmony with the cosmos and the choices to bring that about.

Meditation sets the stage for contact of mind with spirit. By meditation I don't mean Eastern style. I earnestly tried such meditation as a young man—without success; just not for me. I prefer the terms *communing, reflecting,* and *contemplating.* My focused time to commune with my Spirit is when I walk each morning. I reflect upon and discuss my health among many other things. I often come away with an answer of peace, direction, and things to do. I rest, I relax, I commune, I feel better.

Dealing with dementia as a caregiver from a spiritual perspective

I view the purpose of this life as providing favorable conditions that enable the indwelling spirit to grow a soul of nobility, one that survives the grave and games entrance into life never-ending. So growth results from countless moral decisions throughout life in consultation with our highest perception of what God would want in each situation. So it follows that if a person can no longer make moral decisions, then his soul no longer has the capacity to grow. Although the body lives, the soul is in hibernation waiting to be clothed with a new mind and new body in the next life.

What does this mean for dealing with a person who has dementia? It means that you are the caretaker of a body and what remains of the mind. There's no more capacity to grow spiritually and accomplish God's purpose: the creation of a soul that is the joint creation of the human mind and the indwelling divine Spirit. This being the case, I find a divorcement in spirit (there's no longer a spiritual core with which to relate) from the person is needed to create a new relationship. I learned this from experience. I had been the caretaker of my brother from the early stages of his dementia until his death some eight years later. The brother I had known was no longer there; he lost the ability to grow; his soul was asleep.

The point here is that seeing myself as a caretaker of the body and what's left of the mind help me avoid the emotional roller-coaster of caring for a loved one with dementia. While I attempted to honor my brother's wishes and seek his wellbeing as much as he would permit and circumstances allowed, I ignored, circumvented, or refused his wishes that were either not in his best interests or unduly hindered and burdened his caregivers and those with whom he had contact.

This view is useful in evolving a relationship in which you have divorced yourselves from what once was, where free will was sovereign and to be honored. Things change and wisdom dictates changing with them.

Dying with Spiritual Dignity

It is a choice to die with dignity when our days come to an end. Consider these three levels of a dignified death:

- *You* control how and when you die—physical dignity.
- Then there is mental dignity where you refuse to succumb to emotional pleadings to extend your life at any cost. You keep clear minded and emotionally calm.
- Finally there is spiritual dignity. This is where you have an abiding confidence in your life continuing beyond the grave, emerging into life never-ending. It is one without the excruciating pain and horrors so often found here, but rather a life of ongoing challenge and growth in an atmosphere suffused with love.

Looking at the decision from a spiritual perspective, meaning from the viewpoint of maximizing spiritual growth, the question arises: Can the circumstances of a deteriorating physical body augment spiritual growth? Well may you ask, *How can the declining quality of my life—and its increasing focus on my health issues to the exclusion of so much of what my life had been—add to the growth of my soul?*

The answer resides in your personal connection to God Within. Can you hear the *still small voice* speaking to you, giving you comfort, understanding, and guidance? It is difficult in such dire circumstances. But you can know the work of Spirit by the changes you are experiencing. Do you perceive your inner life changing? For example, has your illness caused you to treat others with more empathy and kindness? Do you find yourself valuing relationships with others more than you once did? Are you thankful and grateful for the care and concern you are receiving whereas before you took for granted the ministrations and loving care of others?

These reflect changes of character, an evidence of soul growth. To this end, continuing to deal with the misery, pain, and difficulties of a deteriorating body has value. Keep in mind that oftentimes while undergoing the trials of life they are not recognized for the spiritual growth and strengthened character they bring about. The value of such suffering is recognized only later, after reflecting on how you have changed or been led into a new direction. Think back on your life and you'll no doubt find difficult or even terrible situations that you are now glad to have suffered through because of how your life changed for the better.

Nonetheless, there may come a time to take control and conclude the earthly ordeal of unendurable pain and disease, whether by stopping artificial measures to prolong life or actively doing so (see www.finalexitnetwork.org). Regardless, your spiritual status continues into the next life exactly where it leaves off here. In other words, God will welcome you in his loving embrace and the adventure of eternity.

AFTERWORD

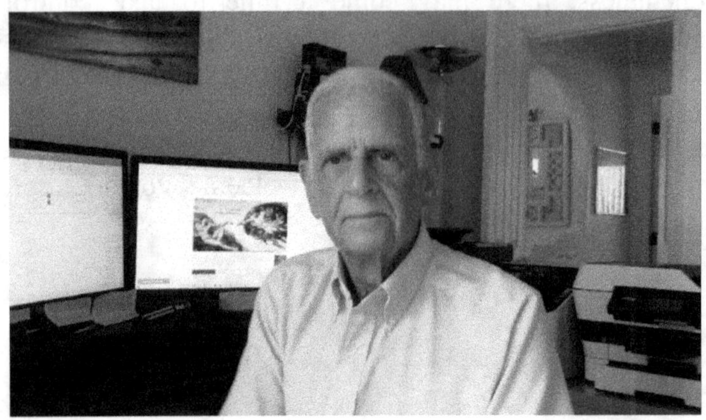

I have laid out my observations about how to optimize health and be wise in dealing with the medical establishment. I covered alternative solutions to be healed and remain healthy. I also reviewed the conventional medical establishment and its limitations. And finally, the integration of physical health with mental clarity and spiritual insight. Without a body that is physically sound, neither mind nor spirit will work as well as it could. And until body, mind, and spirit work in harmony, a person cannot be all that he is purposed to be.

There are more remedies to health problems than you can possibly try; nature abundantly provides for all things. That's why being in touch with your innate guidance system is so important. As with everything in life, we must decide among options. This is where knowledge together with the wisdom of experience comes into play—the result of synchrony with the cosmos and the unity of body-mind-spirit. Achieving optimal health requires us to vigilantly fine-tune and balance the inputs that comprise our physical, emotional, mental, and spiritual wellbeing.

Taking control of your health is not easy with the vast majority of people giving away their sovereignty by uncritically acquiescing to direction from institutional medical authority. It takes courage to retain independent thinking and make your own healthcare decisions. Let such courage be in you.

Checklist

- Commit the time to become knowledgeable about healthy living.
- Eat whole foods (not processed).
- Avoid toxins and toxic environments.
- Learn about and correct your posture.
- Exercise and move.
- Manage stress.
- Reflect carefully about health care decisions.
- Enlist the services of an alternative medicine practitioner.

END NOTES

1 Yun, Dawn. (January 30, 2004). Stroke of inspiration / How Ram Dass sees his nearly fatal attack as a moment of grace. San Francisco Chronicle. https://www.sfgate.com/news/article/Stroke-of-inspiration-How-Ram-Dass-sees-his-2826580.php

2 Hay, William Howard. (1929). Health Via Food. https://www.amazon.com/Health-via-Food-William-Howard-ebook/dp/B00JRGBN9U. Free download at https://soilandhealth.org/wp-content/uploads/02/0201hyglibcat/020165.hay.pdf

3 Levy, Thomas. (2021). Rapid Virus Recovery. Medfox Publishing.

4 The Urantia Book. (1955). 73:6:1 (825.6).

5 Hay, Health Via Food.

6 Ibid.

7 The Guardian. (n.d.). Diversion tactics: how big pharma is muddying the waters on animal antibiotics. https://www.theguardian.com/environment/2018/jun/19/animal-antibiotics-calm-down-about-your-chicken-says-big-pharma

8 Chimonger (username), Registered Nurse and Therapeutic Massage Practitioner. (September 8, 2019). Reinventing Healthcare. www.mercola.com.

9 Mercola, Joseph. (October 10, 2012). Shocking Dangers of Plavix Revealed in 2nd Comparison Study.

Research investigating the effects of Plavix in combination with aspirin versus using aspirin alone for the prevention of stroke and cognitive decline has confirmed previous findings: The combination treatment significantly increases risk of death; doubles risk of gastrointestinal bleeding; and more than doubles fatal hemorrhaging. The anti-platelet arm of the study was terminated as a result of these increased risks to participants.

Plavix when combined with aspirin, the drug nearly doubled the death rate from heart disease among patients who had not had a previous heart attack but were at risk, compared to those taking aspirin alone.

10 Mercola, Joseph. (February 10, 2016). 5 Great Reasons Why You Should Not Take Statins.

[11] Graveline, Duane, M. D. (2006) Lipitor Thief of Memory.

[12] Haag, Myrna. (nd). The Hidden Battle. Myrna Method Clinical Nutrition. https://www.MyrnaMethod.com/

[13] A Midwestern Doctor. (December 25, 2025). Restoring Healthy Relationships at the Dinner Table. https://www.midwesterndoctor.com/i/182558745/healthy-cooking

[14] Mercola, Joseph. (May 18, 2010). Why US Meats Are Horrendous: The Vulgar Truth About What You Eat with that Steak or Burger.

[15] Maurer, Richard. (2014). The Blood Code: Unlock the Secrets of Your Metabolism.

[16] Prouty, Olive Higgins (1941). Now, Voyager.

[17] Mercola, Joseph. (August 3, 2018). Echinacea: The All-American Flower.

[18] Bennet, Carrie. (Aug 30, 2023). Quantum Health 101: What is "Quantum Health?" https://www.carriebwellness.com/blog/quantum-health-101-what-is-quantum-health

[19] Armstrong, Ashley. (N.D.). Why We Don't Believe in Supplement Culture. https://www.youtube.com/shorts/aDS2Bo_qNYk.

[20] A Midwestern Doctor. (January 27, 2025). Making Each of Us Healthy Again. https://www.midwesterndoctor.com/p/making-each-of-us-healthy-again.

[21] Mercola, Joseph. (September 20, 2012). The Diet Doctor Everybody Loves – Gary Taubes.

[22] Shallenberger, Frank. Chelation/CheZone Therapy. https://www.antiagingmedicine.com/treatments/chelation-chezone-therapy-colon-hydrotherapy.

[23] Hertoghe, Thierry. (2002). The Hormone Solution: Stay Younger Longer with Natural Hormone and Nutrition Therapies. New York: Three Rivers Press, p. 118.

[24] Mercola, Joseph. (October 6, 2007). The Greatest Nutrition Researcher of the 20th Century.

[25] Levy, Thomas. (2021). Rapid Virus Recovery. Medfox Publishing.

[26] Staff Report. (April 25, 2014). Alternative Health: Trend or Anomaly? *The Daily Bell*. http://www.thedailybell.com/news-analysis/35246/Alternative-Health-Trend-or-Anomaly/.

[27] Mercola, Joseph. (February 6, 2018). Can the Conventional Medical Profession Be Trusted?

[28] Mercola, Joseph. (September 26, 2018). Billionaire Opioid Executive Stands to Make Millions More on Patent for Addiction Treatment.

[29] Randall, TC. (2010). Forbidden Healing: The Curiously Simple Solution to Disease. Publishing Directions.

[30] Ibid.

[31] Staff Report. (April 29, 2104). Monsanto Meme Disintegrates as Organic Ascends? *The Daily Bell*. http://www.thedailybell.com/news-analysis/35256/Monsanto-Meme-Disintegrates-as-Organic-Ascends/.

[32] Weil, Andrew. (1995). Spontaneous Healing. Ballantine Books. p.59.

[33] Weil, Andrew. (n.d). What's Wrong with Conventional Medicine. https://www.drweil.com/videos-features/videos/conventional-medicine-shortcomings/

[34] Ober, Clinton, Sinatra, Stephen T., & Zucker, Martin. (2010). Earthing: The most important health discovery ever? Laguna Beach, CA. Basic Health Publications, Inc., pp. 38,39.

[35] Sircus, Dr. Mark. (c. 2006) The Terror of Pediatric Medicine (free eBook is available at www.drsircus.com/free-e-book-the-terror-of-pediatric-medicine).

[36] The Disinformation Playbook. (n.d.). Union of Concerned Scientists. https://www.ucsusa.org/our-work/center-science-and-democracy/disinformation-playbook#.W7is1-WZ2Uk.

[37] Lee, Royal, DDS. (1954). Synthetic vs. Natural Vitamins. https://www.seleneriverpress.com/images/pdfs/Synthetic_vs_Natural_Vitamins_by_Royal_Lee.pdf.

[38] Yun, Dawn. (January 30, 2004). Stroke of inspiration / How Ram Dass sees his nearly fatal attack as a moment of grace. San Francisco Chronicle. https://www.sfgate.com/news/article/Stroke-of-inspiration-How-Ram-Dass-sees-his-2826580.php

[39] The Urantia Book. (1955). 110:1.5

[40] Ballantine, Rudolph. (2011). Radical Healing: Integrating the World's Great Therapeutic Traditions to Create a New Transformative Medicine, 2nd edition. Himalayan Institute Press.

[41] D'Ingillo, Donna. (n.d.). Personality, Spirit, Soul and the Transformation of Human Consciousness. www.InstituteChristConsciousness.org

[42] MacDonald-Bayne, M. (1954). Beyond the Himalayas. London: L.N. Fowler & Co. Ltd, p.22.

[43] Singer, Michael. (2007). The Untethered Soul: The Journey Beyond Yourself. New Harbinger Publications. p.47.